Nutrition Care in Nursing Facilities
SECOND EDITION

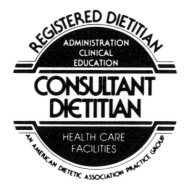

Consultant Dietitians in Health Care Facilities
A Dietetic Practice Group of The American Dietetic Association

Editor-in-Chief
Clara L. Gerwick, RD

Associate Editors
Evelyn S. Hiett, RD
Kathleen C. Niedert, MBA, RD
Mary Ellen Posthauer, RD

THE AMERICAN DIETETIC ASSOCIATION

Library of Congress Cataloging-in-Publication Data

Nutrition care in nursing facilities.—2nd ed./Consultant Dietitians in Health Care Facilities, a dietetic practice group of the American Dietetic Association; Clara L. Gerwick, editor-in-chief; Evelyn S. Hiett, Kathleen C. Niedert, Mary Ellen Posthauer, associate editors.

       p. cm.

     Rev. ed. of: Nutrition in long-term care facilities/ Anna Katherine Jernigan. c1987.

     Includes bibliographical references and index.

     ISBN 0-88091-105-0

     1. Long-term care facilities—Food service—Management. 2. Chronically ill—Nutrition. I. Gerwick, Clara L. II. Jernigan, Anna Katherine. Nutrition in long-term care facilities. III. Consultant Dietitians in Health Care Facilities.

     [DNLM: 1. Dietary Services—handbooks. 2. Long-Term Care—organization & administration—handbooks. 3. Nutrition—in old age—handbooks. 4. Quality Assurance, Health Care—handbooks. QU39 N976]

  RA999.F65J47   1992

  362.1'76'0846—dc20

  DNLM/DLC

  for Library of Congress   92-49942
                                     CIP

Printed in the United States of America.

CONTENTS

FOREWORD

The nutrition needs of the nursing facility resident are presented in this manual. In nursing facilities, nutrition assessments can identify those who could benefit from nutrition support, thus decreasing the costs and debilitating effects of malnutriton.

This manual emphasizes quality care and residents' rights as well as the importance of individualizing nutrition services based on available resources and operating procedures in the institution to meet the needs of each resident.

This focus is congruent with The American Dietetic Association's Strategic Thinking Initiative. This strategic plan promotes member recognition to the public, government, industry, and allied professions as the experts on food and nutrition as they relate to the quality of life. The actions of ADA are to serve the profession best by serving the public first. These actions reflect the following values: excellence, leadership, integrity, respect, and communication.

The Consultant Dietitians in Health Care Facilities (CD-HCF), the oldest and largest practice group of The American Dietetic Association, represents more than 5200 registered dietitians who subscribe to this forward-thinking plan. Our members are committed to improving the nutritional health of the public and providing cost-effective management of foodservice operations.

In keeping with ADA's strategic plan and CD-HCF's purpose, we offer this manual to you, the caregiver, in addressing the nutrition needs of residents in nursing facilities.

Sharon Burns, RD
Chairman, 1991-92
Consultant Dietitians in Health Care Facilities

PREFACE

The American Dietetic Association requested our practice group, Consultant Dietitians in Health Care Facilities, to revise the 1987 handbook, *Nutrition in Long-Term Care Facilities*. We accepted this opportunity with enthusiasm since we as consultant dietitians work in the nursing facility every day and we could provide the current knowledge and practicum to assist others. It has been a tremendous challenge and a rewarding experience.

Therefore, the purpose of this handbook is to provide guidelines for the assessment of the nutritional status of the elderly and the provision of nutrition support. It is not intended to be all-inclusive, but it does provide a compilation of information the registered dietitian needs in providing nutrition care in the nursing facility. Since it is such a fast growing field it should be remembered that information presented here should be reviewed in light of new information as it becomes available.

With the many changes in the nursing facility field, the editorial committee determined that much of the previous manual needed revision including name. Since the industry that represents long-term care facilities now refers to their homes as nursing facilities, we chose the name *Nutrition Care in Nursing Facilities*. Another small change was to identify our clients as "residents" not "patients" because the nursing facility is now their home.

The table of contents was organized in a manner in which the new professional would need the information required to meet the facility needs. For the practicing registered dietitian the chapter identity should provide the clue where to find the required information. Beginning with standards of practice, interventions in malnutrition as it relates to various disease entities, environmental risk factors, professional responsibilities to maintain quality of life, measuring performance of nutrition care, essential determinants needed for completion of the nutrition assessment, enhancing the dining experience, and finally, the individualized care plan are provided. The ultimate goal for the registered dietitian and the other health care team members is to help each resident attain the highest quality of life possible.

To attain the goal we had set for ourselves, I was blessed to have three dedicated, competent, practicing registered dietitians as my committee. They not only edited but wrote a great deal of the following manuscript. I wish to give a very warm personal thank you to Evelyn S. Hiett, RD, consultant dietitian, Littleton, Colorado; Kathleen C. Niedert, MBA, RD, director of nutrition and dining services, Allen Memorial Hospital, Waterloo, Iowa; and Mary Ellen Posthauer, RD, president, M.E.P. Healthcare Services, Inc., Evansville, Indiana.

As a committee we are grateful to our authors. Each is very special in our eyes, and we feel you will share that as you use the manual.

We are very indebted to each of our excellent reviewers for having taken time from their busy schedules to critique the content.

And finally I need to give a warm personal thanks to my office manager, Elaine Long, who did all of the word processing and assisted in numerous other ways. Without her, we would not have made it.

Each of us working in nursing facilities can have a positive impact on each resident as we accept the opportunity to be proactive in assessing the needs of residents, in delivering high quality nutritional care, and in eliminating or reducing malnutrition.

Clara L. Gerwick, RD
C. L. Gerwick and Associates, Inc.
Overland Park, Kansas

ACKNOWLEDGMENTS

On behalf of the Consultant Dietitians in Health Care Facilities, a practice group of The American Dietetic Association, I wish to thank the individuals who so graciously accepted our request to write a chapter or section. It truly was a labor of love from each of them.

Contributors

Ann Moore Allen, MS, RD
Retired Co-author of *Food-Medication Interactions*
Tempe, Arizona

Rosemary Behrens, RD
Executive, Visions for Success
Ossian, Iowa

Anne Kriener Blocker, RD
Executive, Visions for Success
Waukon, Iowa

Johanna T. Dwyer, DSc, RD
Director, Francis Stern Nutrition Center
Professor, Tufts University Schools of Medicine and Nutrition
Senior Scientist, USDA Human Nutrition Research Center on Aging at Tufts University
Boston, Massachusetts

Ann Gallagher, RD
President, F.A. Gallagher and Associates
Fort Wayne, Indiana

Kathleen Pintell, RD
Consultant Dietitian
Butler, Pennsylvania

Jean Inman, MBA, RD
President, The New England Center for Nutrition Education, Inc.
Stoughton, Massachusetts

Vicki Kuzniar, RD
Denver General Hospital
Denver, Colorado

Carlene Russell, MS, RD
Consultant Dietitian
St. Joseph Mercy Hospital
Mason City, Iowa

Jane V. White, PhD, RD
Associate Professor
Department of Family Medicine
University of Tennessee Graduate School of Medicine
Knoxville, Tennessee

Reviewers

Sharon Burns, RD
Consultant Dietitian
Armada, Michigan

Emma Luten, MS, RD
Chief, Survey Training Team
Health Care Financing Administration
Baltimore, Maryland

Kathleen Pintell, RD
Consultant Dietitian
Butler, Pennsylvania

1. STANDARDS OF PRACTICE

The American Dietetic Association Code of Ethics for the Profession of Dietetics

Standards of Practice of the Consultant Dietitians in Health Care Facilities

Liability and Malpractice Insurance

1. STANDARDS OF PRACTICE

The American Dietetic Association
Code of Ethics for the Profession of Dietetics

PREAMBLE

The American Dietetic Association and its credentialing agency, the Commission on Dietetic Registration, believe it is in the best interests of the profession and the public it serves that a Code of Ethics provide guidance to dietetic practitioners in their professional practice and conduct. Dietetic practitioners have voluntarily developed a Code of Ethics to reflect the ethical principles guiding the dietetic profession and to outline commitments and obligations of the dietetic practitioner to self, client, society, and the profession.

The purpose of the Commission on Dietetic Registration is to assist in protecting the nutritional health, safety, and welfare of the public by establishing and enforcing qualifications for dietetic registration and for issuing voluntary credentials to individuals who have attained those qualifications. The Commission has adopted this Code to apply to individuals who hold these credentials.

The Ethics Code applies in its entirety to members of The American Dietetic Association who are Registered Dietitians (RDs) or Dietetic Technicians, Registered (DTRs). Except for sections solely dealing with the credential, the Code applies to all American Dietetic Association members who are not RDs or DTRs. Except for aspects solely dealing with membership, the Code applies to all RDs and DTRs who are not ADA members. All of the aforementioned are referred to in the Code as "dietetic practitioners."

PRINCIPLES

1. The dietetic practitioner provides professional services with objectivity and with respect for the unique needs and values of individuals.

2. The dietetic practitioner avoids discrimination against other individuals on the basis of race, creed, religion, sex, age, and national origin.
3. The dietetic practitioner fulfills professional commitments in good faith.
4. The dietetic practitioner conducts him/herself with honesty, integrity, and fairness.
5. The dietetic practitioner remains free of conflict of interest while fulfilling the objectives and maintaining the integrity of the dietetic profession.
6. The dietetic practitioner maintains confidentiality of information.
7. The dietetic practitioner practices dietetics based on scientific principles and current information.
8. The dietetic practitioner assumes responsibility and accountability for personal competence in practice.
9. The dietetic practitioner recognizes and exercises professional judgment within the limits of his/her qualifications and seeks counsel or makes referrals as appropriate.
10. The dietetic practitioner provides sufficient information to enable clients to make their own informed decisions.
11. The dietetic practitioner who wishes to inform the public and colleagues of his/her services does so by using factual information. The dietetic practitioner does not advertise in a false or misleading manner.
12. The dietetic practitioner promotes or endorses products in a manner that is neither false nor misleading.
13. The dietetic practitioner permits use of his/her name for the purpose of certifying that dietetic services have been rendered only if he/she has provided or supervised the provision of those services.
14. The dietetic practitioner accurately presents professional qualifications and credentials.
    A. The dietetic practitioner uses "RD" or "registered dietitian" and "DTR" or "dietetic technician, registered" only when registration is current and authorized by the Commission on Dietetic Registration.
    B. The dietetic practitioner provides accurate information and complies with all requirements of the Commission on Dietetic Registration program in which he/she is seeking initial or continued credentials from the Commission on Dietetic Registration.
    C. The dietetic practitioner is subject to disciplinary action for aiding another person in violating any Commission on Dietetic Registration requirements or aiding another person in representing himself/herself as an RD or DTR when he/she is not.
15. The dietetic practitioner presents substantiated information and interprets controversial information without personal bias,

recognizing that legitimate differences of opinion exist.

16. The dietetic practitioner makes all reasonable effort to avoid bias in any kind of professional evaluation. The dietetic practitioner provides objective evaluation of candidates for professional association memberships, awards, scholarships, or job advancements.

17. The dietetic practitioner voluntarily withdraws from professional practice under the following circumstances:
    A. The dietetic practitioner has engaged in any substance abuse that could affect his/her practice;
    B. The dietetic practitioner has been adjudged by a court to be mentally incompetent;
    C. The dietetic practitioner has an emotional or mental disability that affects his/her practice in a manner that could harm the client.

18. The dietetic practitioner complies with all applicable laws and regulations concerning the profession. The dietetic practitioner is subject to disciplinary action under the following circumstances:
    A. The dietetic practitioner has been convicted of a crime under the laws of the United States which is a felony or a misdemeanor, an essential element of which is dishonesty, and which is related to the practice of the profession.
    B. The dietetic practitioner has been disciplined by a state and at least one of the grounds for the discipline is the same or substantially equivalent to these principles.
    C. The dietetic practitioner has committed an act of misfeasance or malfeasance which is directly related to the practice of the profession as determined by a court of competent jurisdiction, a licensing board, or an agency of a governmental body.

19. The dietetic practitioner accepts the obligation to protect society and the profession by upholding the Code of Ethics for the Profession of Dietetics and by reporting alleged violations of the Code through the defined review process of The American Dietetic Association and its credentialing agency, the Commission on Dietetic Registration.

The Code of Ethics for the Profession of Dietetics of The American Dietetic Association was adopted by the House of Delegates in October 1987, for implementation January 1, 1989.

Standards of Practice of the Consultant Dietitians in Health Care Facilities

The Consultant Dietitians in Health Care Facilities (CD-HCF) was the first dietetic practice group of The American Dietetic Association to develop standards of practice specifically for its members. The CD-HCF standards were written and validated for consultant dietitians to use in evaluating and monitoring dietary services provided to facilities. These registered dietitians must determine the plan of action for each facility, taking into consideration the criteria outlined in the standards of practice.

The Omnibus Budget Reconciliation Act (OBRA) of 1987 requires each nursing facility to have a quality assurance program in place for the entire facility. Dietary quality assurance is part of the overall plan. The registered dietitian must determine appropriate criteria, objectives, and indicators to demonstrate the quality and effectiveness of dietary services and nutrition care provided for residents. The CD-HCF standards of practice assist the registered dietitian in developing such a program.

OBRA supports the role of the registered dietitian as a member of the interdisciplinary team to evaluate, monitor, recommend, and improve nutrition care to residents of nursing facilities. This congressional mandate empowers residents with the right to expect a high quality of nutrition care. Several sets of regulations—including resident's rights, quality of life, resident assessment, and quality of care—definitely impact the care of residents.

Through OBRA Congress enacted sweeping amendments to the Social Security Act that shift the government's focus to the outcome of resident care in nursing facilities. As part of these outcome-oriented changes, every facility must conduct a "comprehensive, accurate, standardized, reproducible" assessment of nutritional status for each resident at the time of admission, and at least annually thereafter. According to OBRA, facilities must ensure that residents maintain or attain "acceptable parameters" of nutritional status. Hence, nutritional status is a clinical indicator used in the survey and certification process.

The registered dietitian is responsible for the documentation of residents' nutrition problems and identification of strengths that can maintain or improve nutritional status. Once problems are identified, appropriate treatment is implemented. As part of the interdisciplinary team, the registered dietitian helps to develop plans of care that ensure the residents' nutrition needs are met and, when possible, to ensure that independence in eating is maintained.

Changes in the Medicare conditions of participation for nursing facilities and in the survey and certification procedures present a potential for expanded nutrition services. With the Health Care Financing Administration's focus on resident outcomes, nursing facilities have strong incentives to maximize their residents' nutritional status. Surveyors evaluate the adequacy of nutrition services by referring to the incidence and healing of nutrition-related problems among the residents. The registered dietitian's services will meet the obligations under these standards.

The registered dietitian has the obligation to ensure that nutrition needs of all residents are met. Responsibilities must include not only clinical services; dietitians must ensure also that excellent quality food is prepared and served under sanitary conditions.

Last but not least, the registered dietitian has the responsibility to provide the most appropriate nutrition care for residents in a cost-effective manner.

Standards of Practice for Consultant Dietitians in Health Care Facilities

The following standards of practice will enable the registered dietitian to set personal goals.

STANDARD 1

The dietetics practitioner establishes performance criteria, compares actual performance with expected performance, documents results, and takes appropriate action.

Criteria	Documentation
1.1 Studies show that the administrative/professional staff feel the consultant dietitian (CD) is functioning according to stated performance criteria.	1.1 The CD annually prepares a written document listing a plan of work, methods of accomplishment and the desired date of completion.
1.2 Consultation reports are acknowledged by the administration and dietary manager. Follow-up is evident by time lines; completion dates are met on recommendations.	1.2 CD reports are available and acknowledged by administrator and food service director or manager of food and nutrition services.
1.3 The dietetics department complies with all applicable state and federal regulations.	1.3 Copies of recent surveys indicate compliance with regulations. The CD notes problem areas and initiates corrective action.
1.4 The dietetics department uses foodservice forms in the efficient operations of the department.	1.4 The CD evaluates foodservice forms as completed by the dietary manager: employee orientation, employee evaluation, food cost records, temperature records, etc.
1.5 Food quality is evident by measurements conducted in the food dietetics department.	1.5 The CD observes meals as prepared and served: monitors temperatures, tastes the food, and uses the monthly report to comment on the quality of the meal.

STANDARD 2

The dietetics practitioner develops, implements, and evaluates an individual plan for practice based on assessment of consumer needs, current knowledge, and clinical experience.

Criteria	Documentation
2.1 A contract between the CD and the facility specifies a plan for services.	2.1 CD's contract specifies responsiblities of CD and of the facility.
2.2 The menus are coordinated, implemented, and evaluated.	2.2 Menus prepared and evaluated for nutritional adequacy, resident acceptance, therapeutic diets, and costs. The CD provides periodic analysis of menus for nutritional adequacy.
2.3 Products/services are coordinated and evaluated.	2.3 Evidence in CD reports or other documentation that the CD evaluates the meal delivery system, current products/services used and products considered for purchase.
2.4 A system for environmental sanitation is developed, implemented, and evaluated.	2.4 Written reports of periodic sanitation and maintenance procedures are prepared or evaluated by the CD as per the dietetics department policy and procedure manual.

STANDARD 3

The dietetics practitioner, utilizing unique knowledge of nutrition, collaborates with other professionals, personnel, and/or consumers, to integrate, interpreting, and communicate nutrition care principles.

Criteria	Documentation
3.1 Resident is evaluated for physical condition and food acceptance.	3.1 Resident visits are recorded in the weekly/monthly report.
3.2 Nutrition care is evaluated and documented in the resident's medical record.	3.2 The CD writes pertinent information in resident charts at regular intervals. Documentation of conferences with appropriated staff concerning nutrition problems appears in monthly reports.

3.3 Inter/intra departmental communications are developed, coordinated and monitored.

3.3 The dietetics department policy and procedure manual details the method of inter and intra department communication.

3.4 The dietetics department's operations manual is developed, implemented, and reviewed annually.

3.4 The policy and procedure manual of the facility's dietetics department states who prepared the manual and specifies schedule review and revision. Manual contains the organization chart, job descriptions, work schedules, department policies, samples of forms used, and other information as deemed necessary.

3.5 Nutrition resources are available to resident/family, dietary staff, facility staff, and administration.

3.5 Nutrition counseling sessions and recommendations for appropriate activities are documented in the monthly report.

3.6 Unique knowledge of nutrition principles are demonstrated by ongoing community service projects.

3.6 The CD is available for participation in the local chapter of such organizations as the American Heart Association, American Diabetes Association, and American Red Cross.

3.7 Facility/staff education and dietetics department in-service education are developed, implemented, and evaluated.

3.7 The dietetics department's policy and procedure manual details the facility's plan for education of the dietetic staff and the facility staff, and there are documented reports of staff education.

STANDARD 4

The dietetics practitioner engages in lifelong self-development to improve knowledge and skills.

Criteria

4.1 Standards for membership in professional organizations are met.

Documentation

4.1 Provides evidence of membership in The American Dietetic Association and Consultant Dietitians in Health Care Facilities dietetic practice group. Provides evidence of

4.2 Practice is enhanced by improving competency and learning related skills.

4.2 The CD meets continuing education requirements as established by the Commission on Dietetic Registration: attends workshops, professional meetings, seminars, and college classes on dietetics and related skills, (eg, writing, speaking, computers, media, time management).

maintaining status as a registered dietitian.

4.3 Self-assessment to identify professional strengths and weaknesses is conducted.

4.3 The CD has a specific, written plan for professional development, including completion dates for specific goals.

4.4 A personal development style is adopted to enhance professional image.

4.4 The CD, as much as possible, adopts a regular exercise program and consumes an adequate diet.

4.5 High standards of personal and professional ethics.

4.5 The CD compares his/her professional conduct with the Code of Ethics for the Profession of Dietetics.

STANDARD 5

The dietetics practitioner generates, interprets, and uses research to enhance dietetic practices.

Criteria	Documentation
5.1 Daily practices reflect current nutrition and management research and implement results.	5.1 Reference materials on nutrition, food systems, management, and equipment are on file. Evaluation of menus, meal service systems, and nutrition assessments justify implementation of research.
5.2 Resident oriented research will be initiated and evaluated	5.2 CD initiates and evaluates research on the nutritional status of residents. Surveys reflecting resident acceptance of programs are on file.

5.3 New products and current trends will be evaluated and implemented.

5.3 Information on new items and trends are on file. Surveys/questionnaires justifying the implementation of these items and results (eg, increased efficiency) are available.

STANDARD 6

The dietetics practitioner identifies, monitors, analyzes, and justifies the use of resources.

Criteria	Documentation
6.1 Tangible resources for the operation of the department are identified and justified.	6.1 Diet manuals and policy and procedure manuals are on file and in use. Documentation of recommendations are in CD report.
6.2 Current management practices of the facility are analyzed.	6.2 CD documents management studies conducted.
6.3 Department costs are monitored and evaluated.	6.3 CD reports include average care costs from the nursing care industry and recommend plans of action to control departmental costs.

Liability and Malpractice Insurance

With increasing independence of action by individual registered dietitians arises the very real issue of personal and professional liability. This issue is especially important to the consultant dietitian.

The nutrition management of residents is constantly becoming more complex with the continuing development of sophisticated parenteral and enteral feeding technology, calorimetry, physiologically based resident assessments, and evaluation for drug-nutrient interactions. As the science of nutrition develops, the practicing physician becomes increasingly dependent on the knowledge and professional judgment of the registered dietitian. This has markedly increased the scope of practice for all registered dietitians. This increasing scope of practice, while positive from the aspect of professional growth, places the registered dietitian squarely in the liability and malpractice arena.

Many registered dietitians are content with the idea that professional liability insurance carried by the facility provides them with adequate protection. This belief may create a false sense of security for the following reasons:

- Coverage is limited. Usually only on-site or on-duty periods are covered, and then only for those who are considered employees of the facility, not contracted consultants. Coverage frequently does not extend to off-duty hours or volunteer duties even though they are performed in the best interest of the facility. Such coverage also does not extend to well-intended advice or information provided to friends, acquaintances, or other employees. The facility's policy may also cover only those duties specified in the job description. With the rapid growth and increased sophistication of modern dietetics, the job description can be quickly "outgrown" thus placing the registered dietitian at risk for "non-covered" duties.

- Policies are designed to serve the interests of the contracting facility, not the consultant. For example, in an individual malpractice action the insurance company may choose to settle out of court, even when the interests of the consultant may be served best by a hearing or trial. The facility's carrier may also countersue the consultant to recover monetary damage incurred by the company because of the consultant's actions. In these countersuits the consultant could be held personally responsible for all costs associated with the countersuit.

- Facility policies may not cover supplementary expenses incurred by the consultant arising from the action. Thus, inconvenience, lost time, and lost wages are the responsibility of the consultant.

The monetary risk to inadequately insured registered dietitians is potentially enormous. Even though a registered dietitian may not currently have assets to satisfy a judgment, any future assets can be attached to satisfy that judgment long after the malpractice action concludes.

The decision to purchase professional malpractice insurance is a personal one. However, in light of our litigious society, it is strongly recommended that registered dietitians protect themselves by carrying adequate insurance.

Bibliography

Brent J. Setting up your own business. *AORN J.* 1990;1:205–213.

Brooke S. Shopping for liability insurance. *Am J Nurs.* 1989;2;171–172.

Feutz A. Do you need professional liability insurance? *Nurs 91.* 1991;1;56–57.

Guido GW. *Legal Issues in Nursing.* Norwalk, Conn: Appleton and Lange; 1988.

2. RELATIONSHIP BETWEEN NUTRITION AND DISEASE IN THE OLDER PERSON

Nutrition Screening Initiative

Interventions in Malnutrition-Related Causes of Disabilities

2. RELATIONSHIP BETWEEN NUTRITION AND DISEASE IN THE OLDER PERSON

Nutrition Screening Initiative

In 1988, the Administration on Aging cosponsored the Surgeon General's Workshop on Health Promotion and Aging. This historic meeting called for coordinated national efforts to promote nutrition screening and intervention in America.[1]

Research proves that, as we approach the 21st century, the elderly are the single largest demographic group with a disproportionate risk of malnutrition.[2] One of the conclusions of the Department of Health and Human Services report, *Healthy People 2000*, is that "Nutrition is one of the many important factors affecting the health and longevity of older persons. But for many low income and minority older Americans, it may be the most important." [1]

The Department of Health and Human Services report further "called for our nation's health care system to increase nutrition assessment and counseling. . .setting the goal that 75% of primary care providers would give nutrition assessment and counseling or make a referral to qualified dietitians." The report concluded, "dietary modification *can* be achieved through primary care interventions. Dietary assessment, advice, counseling, and follow-up by primary care providers and registered dietitians *are* effective." [1]

This document became the framework of the Nutrition Screening Initiative (NSI). The NSI was launched in May 1990 to promote nutrition screening and better nutrition care for our nation's elderly.

The NSI is a 5-year, multidisciplinary campaign under the leadership of the American Academy of Family Physicians (AAFP), The American Dietetic Association (ADA), and the National Council on the Aging, Inc (NCOA). A blue ribbon advisory committee of more than 30 key organizations and professionals from the fields of nutrition, medicine, and aging also plays an important role in guiding the effort. These groups include health professional organizations, social service organizations, and consumer groups and represent some 37 million members.

Key to the ongoing work of the NSI is the technical review committee, which is composed of leading experts in nutrition and geriatrics.

The Initiative pursues its objectives through the following four basic areas of activity, each of which is guided by a working subcommittee:
1. Research and testing
2. Professional education and development
3. Communication with the public
4. Advocacy of public policies in support of nutrition screening and better nutrition care.[2]

Recognizing the need for creating a shared understanding, the Initiative set the goal of developing a common approach to nutrition screening. This basic approach to screening would be adapted by the professionals working at different points along the continuum of care to the specific needs of the clients or patients.[2]

Early discussions among the leaders of the Initiative helped to clarify the need for multidisciplinary formulation of answers to several key questions:

- What does it mean to be at risk for poor nutritional status?
- What does it mean to be suffering from poor nutritional status?
- What constitutes an approach to nutrition screening that could be useful in a variety of settings?
- What interventions showed enough proof or promise of benefit to warrant routine nutrition screening for the elderly?[2]

The first step undertaken by the Initiative to move to a common view was to commission a comprehensive review of the literature pertaining to the prevalence of nutrition-related problems among older Americans and approaches to nutrition screening and assessment. Johanna Dwyer, DSc, RD, director of the Frances Stern Nutrition Center at Tufts University, conducted the research and drew upon the critical analysis and comments of national geriatrics and nutrition experts. Her research summarized the state of both the science and the practice of nutrition care.

The Initiative then embarked on an aggressive multidisciplinary process involving professionals nationwide to develop consensus papers on risk factors associated with poor nutritional status in older Americans, indicators of poor nutritional status in older Americans, and basic nutrition screening techniques. These papers were drafted by members of the technical review committee and underwent two cycles of review by the entire committee and representatives of AAFP, ADA, and NCOA.[2]

A broadly representative, multidisciplinary group of more than 90 individuals and organizations was invited to participate in a consensus process that began in December 1990. That process culminated in a working conference in April 1991, aimed at achieving consensus on the three papers and discussing and acknowledging useful interventions.

Out of the conference came the beginning of a public awareness tool to help people identify whether they may be at risk for poor nutrition: the "Determine Your Nutritional Health" checklist. In February 1992, the US Senate Aging Subcommittee conducted a public education campaign to alert the public and promote the checklist in popular magazines and newspapers. *The Nutrition Screening Manual for Professionals Caring for Older*

Americans[3] also was prepared subsequent to the 1991 conference. The manual shows how to evaluate a person's nutritional status, and the level I and level II screens.

Goals for Change

In summary, the NSI continues to pursue multidisciplinary approaches to:

- Promote and expand existing quality nutrition screening in the nation's health care system.
- Move to incorporate the widespread use of nutrition screening in health and medical care settings.
- Develop and work through a network of dietitians, physicians, health and medical care professionals, aging experts, and others.
- Expand educational outreach to medical and health care professionals, the public, and policy makers.
- Generate additional research on the efficacy and cost effectiveness of nutrition assessments.
- Encourage public policy initiatives in support of nutrition screening and better nutritional care.
- Communicate through mass media to increase public awareness.[4]

References

1. *Healthy People 2000: National Health Promotion and Disease Prevention Objectives.* Washington, DC: US Dept of Health and Human Services; 1990.
2. *Executive Summary, Report of Nutrition Screening 1: Toward a Common View.* Washington, DC: Nutrition Screening Initiative, 1991.
3. *Nutrition Screening Manual for Professionals Caring for Older Americans.* Washington, DC: Nutrition Screening Initiative; 1991.
4. *A Vital Sign of America's Health.* Washington, DC: Nutrition Screening Initiative, 1991.

Interventions in Malnutrition-Related Causes of Disabilities

Aging is the sum of many different biological and psychological changes that occur from birth onward. These occur at rates that vary from person to person. Thus, chronologic age is not descriptive of true functional or biological age.[1-3] Environmental influences also play a role. More people reach older ages today, and those who do are healthier and better nourished at ages 65, 75 and 85 than they were 50 or 100 years ago.

Obesity

DEFINITION

Obesity is usually present when weight exceeds 120% of desirable weight for height as stated in the Metropolitan Life Insurance Company tables of 1983.[4] Obesity is also defined as a body mass index (BMI) in excess of 27.8 for men or 27.3 for women. Severe obesity is a BMI greater than 30.

Standards of weight and body composition by frame size and height are now available for people up to age 74 based on the National Health and Nutrition Examination Survey II.[5] Estimates of obesity at advanced age are difficult because standards are not available. Body composition is different; the contributions of water, the mineral skeleton, and lean body mass to weight are probably less than they were at younger ages.

REASON FOR CONCERN

Many older residents are obese, and others become so as they grow older. Severe obesity contributes to increased mortality. Moderate obesity is associated with increased mortality among the elderly in some studies but not in others, and is currently the topic of much debate.

Severe obesity complicates the health care and nursing of the elderly. Obese elderly residents in nursing facilities have difficulty transferring from bed to chair, may have trouble walking, and find toileting hazardous. They are often prone to falls, and when falls do occur, hip fracture, broken wrists, and cracked vertebrae are common, especially among those who are already osteoporotic. When urinary or fecal incontinence is present and the person is obese, hygiene becomes even more difficult. Among residents who are obese or bed-bound, pressure ulcers, hypostatic congestion of the lungs, and leg vein thromboses are common.

WELL-SUPPORTED INTERVENTIONS

The best intervention ensures that older people never become obese. However, among residents who are already obese, weight reduction is desirable. But very severe restriction of energy intake makes little sense for residents in nursing facilities. Among elderly obese residents who are asymptomatic, the goal is to maintain weight at current levels and to maximize quality of life.

If obese older residents have acute symptoms that might be ameliorated by dietary measures, a more activist stance is warranted, but again, moderation is in order. For example, an obese diabetic resident who has consistently high blood sugar levels and symptoms should lose a small amount of weight. A 1500-kcal diet for women, and an 1800 to 2000-kcal diet for men is a reasonable beginning.

Energy intakes are often already quite low. Small decreases in calories of a constant nature are the most helpful to minimize losses of lean body mass and to avoid a sense of deprivation. Elderly residents often have difficulty gaining back lean body mass once they have lost it, and they may already be taking many medications that may interact and cause side effects.

Diabetes Mellitus

DEFINITION

The two major forms of diabetes are type I, insulin-dependent diabetes mellitus (IDDM), and type II, non-insulin-dependent diabetes mellitus (NIDDM). The vast majority of elderly people with diabetes suffer from NIDDM. Frank diabetes mellitus is indicated by a random plasma glucose level of 200 mg/dL or greater, or a fasting plasma glucose level of 150 mg/dL or more after fasting. However, the levels used to define abnormality in elderly residents are somewhat arbitrary. In practice, diagnostic levels vary a good deal from physician to physician. Some feel that as a rule of thumb after age 60, 10 mg/dL should be added for each decade to standards before declaring diabetes to be present.[6]

REASONS FOR CONCERN

About 8% of all people over 65 in this country have diabetes mellitus, one of the leading causes of disability and death in older adults. Its treatment costs billions of dollars a year, in addition to the considerable human costs of the disease. Several complications and consequences of diabetes in older residents have negative effects on independent functioning. Diabetic retinopathy and cataracts often cause poor vision and blindness; peripheral vascular disease and circulatory disorders cause difficulties walking and sometimes require leg amputations. Small blood vessel disease in diabetes often leads to the nephropathy of diabetes and eventually to end-stage kidney disease and the need for dialysis or transplantation. Other complications include peripheral neuropathy, hypertension, impotence, and especially in uncontrolled disease, cognitive impairment.

WELL-SUPPORTED INTERVENTIONS

In older residents, more than 90% of all diabetes is type II, or NIDDM. The incidence of type II diabetes and its complications increases with age. Both types of diabetes require nutrition therapy. However, quality of life and function must be carefully weighed in devising appropriate action. Foremost is the need to maintain a balanced diet, while avoiding acute symptoms stemming from hypoglycemia or hyperglycemia. Measures to achieve strict definitions of normoglycemia that might be perfectly appropriate in a young person may be out of place, especially in asymptomatic residents. The decision to tolerate blood sugar levels in an elderly resident that may be less than ideal is best made by the physician in consultation with the registered dietitian after taking into account all the health realities of the resident.

Glucose tolerance often declines as people grow older, probably because pancreatic beta cell sensitivity to ingested carbohydrate decreases. At the same time, peripheral resistance to insulin-stimulated glucose disposal rises, owing to the presence of obesity, decreased physical activity, and various chronic diseases.[7] At least one-third of all NIDDM in patients older than 70 years is associated with obesity. Thus, much NIDDM can be prevented or controlled by measures that avoid diabetogenic drugs, decrease obesity, and increase physical activity to the extent possible for the resident. If healthier weight is achieved and excessive weight gain is avoided, the metabolic abnormalities often decrease, drug doses may be lessened, and complications of diseases associated with impaired glucose tolerance may decrease. Healthy, nonobese, physically active residents exhibit relatively modest declines in glucose tolerance with age everywhere in the world. The prevention or control of obesity may lessen manifestations of symptomatic diabetes in older residents.

After instituting moderate measures to reduce body weight, some practitioners adjust dietary intake to decrease dietary saturated fat and increase complex carbohydrate in the diet. Decreasing fat intake, particularly that of saturated fat, helps to lower diet-related risks of coronary artery disease and its complications. Diets that are relatively high in carbohydrate (45% to 65% of total calories) also may increase glucose utilization.[8] Whenever possible, without undue restrictions, it is preferable to lower blood sugar by dietary measures even if hypoglycemic drugs are also used, since it may reduce both the possibilities of side effects and the medication costs.

Some elderly residents with type I (IDDM) diabetes actually have type II diabetes, but were prescribed insulin earlier in their lives. For them, regimens that are more liberal than usual for persons with IDDM may provide sufficient control. Diet, insulin, and physical activity all must be monitored and controlled to prevent acute complications.

Hypertension

DEFINITION

Systolic blood pressure of 160 mm Hg or greater and diastolic pressure less than 90 mm Hg define isolated systolic hypertension. Mixed systolic-diastolic hypertension is indicated by a diastolic pressure of 90 mm Hg or greater coupled with elevated systolic pressures as just defined. Diastolic pressures of 90 to 104 signify mild diastolic hypertension; 105 to 114, moderate; and 115 mm Hg or more indicate severe diastolic hypertension.[9]

REASON FOR CONCERN

More than 60% of all Americans older than 65 years have systolic blood pressures equal to or greater than 140 mm Hg and diastolic pressures of 90 mm Hg—levels that are associated with increased morbidity and mortality in older people. Even more moderate elevations in diastolic blood pressures may increase risks, and it is possible that smaller increases in systolic pressures may also be risky.[10]

High blood pressure is a powerful risk factor for stroke and other cardiovascular disease. High systolic blood pressures are highly correlated with risk of disease and mortality from cardiovascular disease among middle aged and older people. In fact, more than one third of all the strokes in elderly men and more than two thirds in elderly women are directly attributable to hypertension. Because cerebrovascular disease is the third most common cause of morbidity and mortality in people older than 50 years of age, reducing it by any means will provide health gains.

Finally, hypertension is also a risk factor for coronary artery disease. Heart disease is the major cause of death in older people, so reduction in high blood pressure levels will be positive in this respect as well. The mechanisms that stimulate hypertension in older residents probably involve changes relating to both age and disease.[11]

WELL-SUPPORTED INTERVENTIONS

The type and choice of treatment depend on the degree of hypertension, other coexisting morbidities, and resident preferences. Evidence indicates that severe diastolic hypertension in the elderly can be treated effectively. Treatment also has positive effects for mild diastolic hypertension and possible systolic hypertension in older adults.

To help minimize drug doses, moderate sodium restriction may be beneficial for residents in nursing facilities. It is best to focus on moderate sodium restrictions by such means as not adding salt, or to strive for mild restrictions of 2.5 to 4 g. Extremely low sodium diets are unpalatable to most elderly residents.

Older residents often respond well to diuretics, so they frequently constitute the first drug of choice. Potassium supplementation may be necessary if potassium-wasting diuretics are used. Also, low serum potassium levels may develop in residents who take cardiac glycosides. Appropriate potassium supplementation helps to avoid hypokalemia and attendant risks of cardiac arrhythmias. Fortunately, potassium-sparing diuretics are available.

The side effects of antihypertensive medications include hyponatremia, hypokalemia, depression, confusion, and possibly postural hypotension. They are more common in residents older than 75—those who have several other health problems, and who take many medications—than in the younger elderly.[12]

Modification of sodium intake has a place in the management of hypertension, but the effects vary from resident to resident. Not every resident responds to sodium restriction by a drop in blood pressure. Nevertheless, even among those whose blood pressure is sodium-responsive, an alternative for controlling sodium stores in the body can be the use of diuretics. Severely restricting sodium intakes may cause problems for many residents. In some elderly residents, especially the very frail, sodium restriction may produce adverse effects on fluid and electrolyte balance, symptomatic postural hypotension, and hyponatremia or alterations in renal function. Diet palatability also is often poor. Across the board, low sodium prescriptions are outdated. It is important to evaluate each resident separately.

Other ions such as calcium or chloride also may influence blood pressure regulation.[13] In epidemiologic studies, low calcium intakes are associated with increased blood pressures. The utility of calcium supplements or chloride restriction for treatment of hypertension is not established. However, calcium intakes at levels recommended in the current Recommended Dietary Allowances are appropriate.

Hyperlipidemia

DEFINITION

After an extensive review of the literature, the Adult Treatment Panel of the National Cholesterol Education Program classified plasma cholesterol levels below 200 mg/dL as desirable, 200 to 239 mg/dL as borderline, and over 240 mg/dL as high risk. These levels are not specific for age, sex, or race. Subjects in the borderline category were at high risk if they had two or more of the following characteristics: male sex, smoking, diabetes mellitus, hypertension, cerebrovascular or peripheral vascular disease, family history of premature (ie, prior to age 55 years) heart disease, and low (ie, less than 35 mg/dL) high density lipoprotein cholesterol.

REASON FOR CONCERN

The issue of appropriate serum cholesterol levels for residents in the eighth and ninth decades of life is still debated. Little evidence exists as to appropriate levels. At the same time, the issue of very low serum cholesterol levels (below 160 mg/dL) as a sign of possible malnutrition also must be considered.

Elevated serum cholesterol occurs in both males and females as they get older, rising by about 45% in women and 30% in men between their early twenties and their early sixties.[14] These increases are associated with increases in coronary artery disease and death. Menopause usually leads to elevated serum cholesterol values and to increased risk of coronary artery disease. Serum cholesterol rises with age seemingly because of increased production of low density lipoprotein (LDL) cholesterol together with a decreased ability of the body to metabolize and get rid of LDL cholesterol. A possible reason is that there are fewer LDL cholesterol receptors in the liver, in addition to diminished expression of the receptors.[15, 16]

Some elderly nursing facility residents have little interest in their serum cholesterol levels, while others have an obsessive, almost morbid fascination with them. Physicians vary in the approaches they prescribe for elderly residents. For most intensive diet therapy is not recommended. The registered dietitian needs to exercise sound clinical judgment when recommending a strict fat-controlled diet for a high-risk resident, particularly because adequate calorie and protein intake may be a greater problem than fat intake.

WELL-SUPPORTED INTERVENTIONS

Reducing intakes of fat, especially of saturated fat, and cholesterol in young and middle-aged people who are at high risk of heart disease is helpful. There is less evidence available on the positive effects of such changes in older people.[17] Serum cholesterol levels are less predictive of coronary artery disease risks among people over age 65 than they are in younger people.[18] However, lowering serum cholesterol levels in older people may still be beneficial.

For residents aged 70 and older, the benefits of extensive dietary modifications to alter serum lipids are unclear. If such changes involve radical shifts in usual eating habits, the resident may become needlessly anxious; dietary intakes may fall, and quality of life may decline. As with other modifications in diet, food as a source of enjoyment, and the need to keep weight at normal levels are relevant considerations. A reasonable approach is to monitor serum cholesterol, and if levels are elevated, dietary modification may be in order. First and foremost should be the duty to provide a liberalized diet that promotes quality of life.

Elderly residents in nursing facilities sometimes exhibit very low (below 160 mg/dL) serum cholesterol levels, often coupled with low serum albumin, hemoglobin, and hematocrit values. Low serum cholesterol may result from a variety of disease processes or to undernutrition.

Osteoporosis

DEFINITION

Osteoporosis is a disease of the bone in which the bone tissue itself appears to be relatively normal, but there is very little of it. Loss of bone from the skeleton reduces bone strength and increases the likelihood of fractures. Certain stages of life or physical conditions are associated with the onset of osteoporosis; postmenopausal osteoporosis, and involutional or senile osteoporosis in old age; or secondary to other diseases in both women and men. Reduced bone density is often a key factor in diagnosing subclinical osteoporosis. Characteristic fractures—those of the wrist, spine, and hip— and scoliosis also signal its presence. Alterations in posture, loss of height, and changes in physical appearance may also be a consequence of osteoporosis.

REASON FOR CONCERN

Bone mass decreases with advancing age. Symptomatic osteoporosis is like an iceberg, with much undetected asymptomatic disease lying below the surface.[19] Bone loss takes place in both sexes, although faster and from a lower starting mass in women than in men. Small women are particularly prone to the condition. Compact cortical bone in the vertebrae, hands, feet, ribs, hip, and long bones of the appendicular skeleton, accounts for more than three fourths of the weight of the skeleton. It and the spongier trabecular bone of the axial skeleton, flat bones, and ends of long bones both decline. Fractures decrease life expectancy in elderly persons. Attendant disabilities are frequently present: pressure ulcers, pneumonia, urinary tract infections, and depression. Those problems, in turn, increase dependence and restrict activity.

WELL-SUPPORTED INTERVENTIONS

Preventive measures earlier in life, including proper diet, can influence bone density of the skeleton and, hence, reduce the risk of fracture. Nutrition can alter the risk of osteoporosis through its effects on bone density. Both peak bone mass and the subsequent loss of bone can be influenced by nutritional factors. The peak bone mass achieved depends on genetics, sex, physical activity, and intakes of calcium-rich foods in childhood, adolescence, and young adulthood. Subsequent bone loss is also affected by nutritional factors, including calcium intake and adequacy of vitamin D.

The most effective preventive measure to decrease loss of bone at the menopause is hormone replacement therapy and consumption of at least the Recommended Dietary Allowance (RDA) for calcium, phosphorus, and vitamin D, coupled with regular exercise.

Hormone replacement therapy cannot prevent bone loss that is often present in extreme old age in both sexes, and it is not effective in preventing secondary osteoporosis due to other causes. However, some physicians prescribe low doses of hormone replacement therapy to very elderly residents, even though its effectiveness in slowing either osteoporosis or heart disease is unknown. Nutritional measures help prevent some forms of osteoporosis associated with extreme age. Senile osteoporosis is sometimes due in part to low intakes of calcium that generate a secondary hyperparathyroidism. Therefore both men and women should consume RDA levels of calcium. Many elderly people avoid milk and milk products. Because these are the major sources of calcium and vitamin D in American diets, their intake of these nutrients may be too low. Calcium intakes must cover both obligatory outputs in the urine, feces, and sweat each day; otherwise, bone mineral stores of the nutrient will be depleted to maintain serum calcium levels.

Decline in calcium absorption associated with aging also plays a role in this form of osteoporosis. Calcium absorption decreases with age; even if the amount of calcium in the diet remains constant, sufficient amounts of it may not reach body cells if intakes fail to meet RDA levels, currently 800 mg per day.

Some residents have inadequate intakes of vitamin D or changes in the metabolism of vitamin D, so vitamin D intakes are also of concern.[20] Skin synthesis of the vitamin from pro vitamin D declines with age, sunlight exposure is often low, and many older people use sun blocks that effectively screen out the ultraviolet rays necessary to convert pro vitamin D into biologically active vitamin D in the skin. Also, the malabsorption of fat and fat-soluble vitamin D, liver disease, kidney disease, and certain other diseases also alter the metabolism of vitamin D.[21] In northern latitudes such as the New England states, vitamin D exposure during winter is so low that calcium metabolism is compromised and bone density decreases in some residents.[22] Therefore, it is important to stress the need to consume at least the RDA for vitamin D, which is currently 5 μg per day. Residents who cannot tolerate food sources of the vitamin may need to take a supplement. Supplements of 400 IU vitamin D are known to be safe; doses greater than 1000 IU per day are not recommended.

Elderly residents who are chronic alcoholics and smokers also increase their risks for osteoporosis. Abstinence may not reverse the course of the disease, but may retard it. In any event, there are other health reasons for moderation in these respects.

Weight-bearing exercise, especially walking and aerobics, may increase bone formation and strengthen muscles so that falls are less likely. Exercise is thus a preventive and curative measure.

Secondary osteoporosis results from many different diseases and can be induced by some drugs.[23] Common diseases and conditions include kidney disease, hyperthyroidism, chronic obstructive pulmonary disease, and post-thyroidectomy and post-gastrectomy status.[24] Drugs that may increase bone loss include steroids, anticonvulsants (eg, phenobarbital and dilantin), and many others. Aluminum-containing antacids also wash out bone if prescribed injudiciously. People with these conditions need monitoring since they are at high risk.

Nutrition intervention is imperative to meet the increased energy and nutrient needs of the elderly resident after fracture. Adequate nutrition coupled with rehabilitation therapy lessens risk for pneumonia and the wasting that often ensues with prolonged immobilization.[25,26]

Chronic Obstructive Pulmonary Disease

DEFINITION

Chronic obstructive pulmonary disease (COPD) is a slow, progressive, disabling condition involving chronic airflow obstruction. It is usually due to chronic bronchitis, emphysema, or other lung disease. People with COPD commonly suffer from cough, dyspnea, generalized difficulty in breathing, wheezing, and increased sputum production. The most common causes of the condition are chronic emphysema and bronchitis due to cigarette smoking and the late effects of respiratory illnesses earlier in life. Asthma usually is not included in considerations of COPD.

REASON FOR CONCERN

A major cause of death and functional limitation in older residents, COPD is the fourth leading cause of death in people older than 65. It is second only to coronary artery disease as a cause of Social Security compensation for disability.[27] Without treatment, patients will most likely experience declines in functional ability, frequent hospitalization, loss of independence, and decreased quality of life. Appetite is often poor. The disease itself and side effects of medications such as theophylline and steroids may cause poor appetite or anorexia. The anorexia may be so severe that protein-energy malnutrition ensues, leading to further declines in pulmonary muscle function. As COPD progresses, respiratory inefficiency increases, and infections, often with fever, are more common, causing energy needs to rise at the very time food intake and appetite are falling, thus intensifying the undernutrition.[28] When exertion is difficult, energy output from physical activity falls but the reduced output is inadequate to compensate for other increases in energy needs. Unless nutrition support is provided, residents in respiratory failure may become even more malnourished when they are given ventilator support.

WELL SUPPORTED INTERVENTIONS

First, it is vital for residents with COPD who also smoke, to stop. Even after COPD has begun to develop, cessation of smoking will decrease rate of loss of lung function. Smoking can also trigger asthma, further complicating treatment.[29] Also, smoking has anorectic effects in many residents, making nutritional rehabilitation difficult. Rehabilitation must address multiple aspects of breathing problems. Drug therapy, exercise, and reconditioning are all thought to improve quality of life and to reduce hospitalizations. Vaccination with pneumonia and influenza vaccines is a high priority since lung function is poor. Comprehensive respiratory care helps maintain functional independence, although it cannot reverse lung damage. Within this total context of care, nutrition is also important.

Many residents with COPD are emaciated. Further weight loss often occurs as the disease progresses. The more severe the airway obstruction, the more nutritional status is likely to deteriorate.[30,31] The cause of increased energy needs among residents with COPD is unclear. Probably the greater respiratory inefficiency increases resting energy expenditures.[32-34] The more malnourished the resident becomes, the more resting energy requirements appear to rise. This may be due to increased need for augmenting ventilation because of reduced ventilatory muscle efficiency, or because of an association between severe COPD and malnutrition. Energy expenditure increases greatly during physical activity, with respiratory infections, and with disease progression. Thus, special nutrition support measures may be necessary.[35-37] Cyanotic residents, sometimes referred to as "blue bloaters" because of their appearance, are especially likely to be malnourished. They are usually hypoxemic, and suffer from secondary polycythemia, carbon dioxide retention, and cor pulmonale.

Residents with weight loss deserve particular attention, since suboptimal body weight is associated with increased morbidity and mortality.[38] Because residents in nursing facilities usually have advanced disease, some weight loss may have already occurred. It is most productive to intervene with nutrition support when weight loss begins. Calorie-dense meals and supplements are helpful. Small, frequent meals are tolerated better than a few large meals. Studies have shown that during large meals, oxygen saturation may fall, producing severe shortness of breath. Adequate fluid intake, including hot drinks and soups, helps to loosen secretions and promote mucus clearance and can also help to add nutrients. It is important to check medications in residents who complain of anorexia. If medications causing anorexia are being used, consider lower doses or alternative drugs. Nutrition rehabilitation may improve respiratory and skeletal muscle function, strength, endurance and work efficiency, and generally improve quality of life.[39]

Malnutrition and weight loss often accompany acute episodes of illness, especially those involving respiratory failure. Both the disease and the accompanying inanition further weaken respiratory muscles and control over ventilation.[40,41] Dyspnea in elderly residents with COPD is further complicated by coexisting conditions, such as congestive heart failure, interstitial lung disease, and pulmonary emboli. All of these conditions may require treatment with medications that further decrease appetite, thereby complicating nutrition therapy and necessitating the use of supplements and enteral or parenteral nutritional support.[42]

Residents who have suffered a great deal of weight loss already and are in end-stage COPD benefit less from supplementary feeding than those who are treated earlier in the disease and at earlier stages of undernutrition.

Increases in metabolic demand with refeeding are often poorly tolerated, and neither respiratory nor skeletal muscle functions improve significantly.[43,44] The diaphragm muscles may be further weakened due to malnutrition, increasing muscle failure, fatigue, and the likelihood of ventilatory compromise with even greater increase in risk of infections. Malnutrition may also compromise the immune system, further predisposing the resident to infections. All of these changes probably account for the worsened survival observed among malnourished COPD residents.[45]

In acutely ill COPD residents, pulmonary insufficiency may be worsened by feedings that contain large amounts of carbohydrate. Carbohydrate generates greater amounts of carbon dioxide in oxidation than does protein or fat. Thus, with high carbohydrate feedings, resting energy expenditure and the thermic response to food tend to be elevated at least to some extent, although not as much as they are in malnourished residents without COPD.[46] Such increases further complicate the refeeding task. Special supplements and feedings low in carbohydrate may be helpful in such residents, particularly those who are on ventilators.

Other residents, sometimes referred to as "pink puffers" (because of their flushed appearance, breathlessness, hyperinflation, mild hypoxemia, and low Pco_2) are sometimes obese. Obese residents need special attention in obtaining a balanced nutrient intake, especially if they need to lose weight. Protein-energy malnutrition has the same ill effects among the obese as it does among the underweight.

Nutrition support of COPD residents needs to start early in the disease, before weight loss and other symptoms become severe. In nursing facilities, residents usually are suffering from advanced disease already. High caloric density, low carbohydrate, increased fat feedings may help improve ventilation. Special formulas may be helpful in achieving these aims. Dietary measures should be coupled with a comprehensive program of therapy and rehabilitation.

Cancers

DEFINITION

Cancer is an inclusive term for a variety of malignant neoplastic diseases. Cancer cells have little or no constraint on new growth and thus are termed neoplastic. They are usually malignant, meaning that they tend to grow progressively more uncontrolled, invading other cells, and causing death unless successfully treated. Many cancers can be cured if they are detected and treated promptly.

REASON FOR CONCERN

Some forms of cancer appear to be associated with diet, but many other risk factors are also involved. However, in spite of advances in knowledge, many gaps still remain, and at present diet-related advice is based on prudent guesses, not on certainties.[47]

Cancer is a disease associated with aging. Total cancer incidence rises with age, with the most common sites after age 65 being the lung, breast, ovaries, prostate, colon, rectum, and pancreas.[48] During the last half century, age-adjusted lung cancer rates have risen, stomach cancer rates have fallen, and the incidence of other cancers has remained fairly stable, although mortality rates for some other cancers have declined. Cancer still accounts for about 20% of all deaths among the elderly. Early intervention is effective in many forms of cancer.

The incidence of malnutrition is high among residents with advanced cancers, particularly among those suffering from cancers of the alimentary tract. Protein-energy malnutrition is the most common secondary diagnosis in such cancers, and it frequently contributes to the cause of death. Metabolic aberrations due to the cancer may accelerate the rate of malnutrition.[49] The prognosis for undernourished residents is poor. It is not yet clear in which types of cancer aggressive nutrition support to reverse or prevent weight loss can improve survival.[50]

WELL SUPPORTED INTERVENTIONS

The registered dietitian's first task in dealing with residents with cancer is to establish rapport and put their minds at ease. Many residents believe that their cancers are due to foods they ate in the past. While diet may play a role in the causation of certain cancers, there is virtually no evidence that diet alone, excluding other risk factors, causes or cures cancer.[51] Many unsubstantiated nutrition remedies are advertised that falsely claim to reverse the course of the disease, and some elderly residents fall victim to well-meaning but uninformed advocates of "nutritional cures" such as vitamins, health foods, and special diets (macrobiotics, vegetarian diets, fasting, and coffee enemas).[52-54] Dietary advice and guidance may help minimize the use of questionable diets and nutritional remedies.

The second task confronting the registered dietitian is to remember that all stress, including the stress of cancer and its therapy, tend to affect older people more than younger people, and that the elderly take longer to recover. Five-year survivals for most forms of cancer decrease with advancing age. Thus additional dietary counseling and nutrition support are needed to minimize preventable adverse effects.

There are no nutrition therapies that can cure cancer in and of themselves. For this we must rely on treatments such as surgery, chemotherapy, radiation, and immunotherapy. Responses are often good in elderly residents, so age alone is no contraindication to treatment. However, these treatment modalities, along with psychological factors such as depression associated with diagnosis and therapies, probably contribute to malnutrition.[55] Therefore a nutrition care plan and continued surveillance are mandatory. The effectiveness of cancer therapy is sometimes hampered by malnutrition. For example, complications of radiation-induced enteritis may result in cessation of radiation therapy in bladder cancer, thereby diminishing the effectiveness of potentially curative therapy and negatively influencing long-term prognosis.[56] Some evidence exists that less nausea and vomiting are associated with chemotherapy in older than in younger persons. Nevertheless, it is important to keep the resident well hydrated so that dehydration will not result if vomiting occurs. Some residents also suffer from constipation as a side effect of some forms of chemotherapy.

All cancer residents deserve nutrition care.[57-59] The most appropriate dietary alterations for managing residents with cancer depends on the underlying pathology of the organ systems affected, the stage of the illness, and other treatments being administered. Therefore, it is important to tailor dietary modifications and nutrition support techniques to the resident's unique situation. Nutrition support is useful during active antitumor therapy if the resident is likely to lose significant weight, is losing weight progressively, or has already lost weight. Dietary counseling and nutrition support involving special supplements are often needed once the resident completes cancer therapy if he or she is in a debilitated state. Residents who fail to gain weight postoperatively do not always have metastatic disease; sometimes they simply are not consuming adequate dietary intakes. Vigilance coupled with long-term nutrition intervention and monitoring help maximize nutritional status. For all residents, oral or enteral feedings are preferable to parenteral feeding whenever possible because of fewer complications. Nasogastric and tube feedings with pumps help when anorexia or dysphagia prevent adequate oral feeding. Usually if the length of time is more than 7 to 14 days, gastrostomy tubes or other methods are considered in place of nasogastric tubes, to maintain quality of life better.

Parenteral and enteral nutrition may enable residents to survive toxic chemotherapy and bone marrow transplantation.[60,61] Nutrition intervention helps residents overcome treatable consequences of cancer therapy that otherwise predispose them to nutrition problems.

Although there is no assurance that providing better nutrition or parenteral or enteral support improve overall clinical outcomes, we do know that malnutrition has a negative impact on prognosis.[62] The basic problem seems to be that at later stages of some forms of cancer, malnutrition is secondary to metastatic disease and is not amenable to intervention by nutritional means.[63]

Indications for special enteral and parenteral nutritional support are published by the American Society of Parenteral and Enteral Nutrition.[64] In elderly residents suffering from cancer, difficult clinical and ethical decisions must be made before starting such therapy. One expert concluded that "nutrition support is contraindicated if the risks exceed the potential benefits, and the consent of the resident or the legal surrogate is required. Because artificially supplied nutrition can protract the terminal phase of many illnesses, withholding or withdrawing nutrition support can be a major ethical and legal problem, especially in incompetent and institutionalized residents."[65] The resident, family, and health care professionals must examine the benefits and burdens of the different feeding modalities; then, they can make reasoned and compassionate decisions.[66]

Enteral feeding may still be appropriate for a resident who is not a candidate for antitumor therapy, if the resident agrees, if the resident has a functional gastrointestinal tract, and if the benefits outweigh the burdens.

Even when a resident is terminally ill with cancer, food and drink are appropriate as palliative measures to promote comfort, overcome bothersome symptoms, and perhaps, improve cosmetic appearance, quality of life, and function.[67]

Renal Disease

DEFINITION

Chronic renal disease is diminution in kidney function severe enough to produce biochemical abnormalities and a decrement in glomerular filtration rate (GFR). Chronic renal failure refers to the clinical condition that results from chronic renal disease, owing to a build-up of waste products and abnormal blood chemistry associated with decline in kidney function. Acute renal failure may result from trauma or other causes, and has similar hallmarks, but it is often reversible.

REASON FOR CONCERN

As people age, their kidney function alters. Changes sometimes involve decreased renal blood flow, decreased GFR, and impaired handling of water and electrolytes. Other problems may involve the metabolism of vitamin D, responsiveness to antidiuretic hormone, and alterations in the renin-angiotensin system.[68] In spite of these changes, kidney function in most older people is usually satisfactory with no apparent clinical signs or symptoms. However, reserve capacity is affected. For example, urine concentrating ability may decrease, so that obligatory water losses are increased after a large solute load, just as they are in young infants.

When concurrent disease or severe stresses are also present in an elderly person, renal problems may arise. Many different pathologic processes lead to deranged and insufficient renal regulatory and excretory function. Among the most common diseases in older individuals with implications for the kidney are chronic glomerulonephritis, hypertension, atherosclerotic cardiovascular disease, diabetes mellitus, some cancers, drug and medication toxicities, untreated prostatic hypertrophy, congestive heart failure, and volume depletion resulting in prerenal azotemia.

Regardless of the cause of the kidney disease, when GFR decreases by 50% or more, declines in renal function continue in a progressive and more or less linear fashion until end-stage renal disease ensues. At this point, dialysis or transplantation are the only alternative to death.

WELL-SUPPORTED INTERVENTIONS

Nutrition interventions currently are being studied for their possible utility early in the course of chronic progressive renal disease, before symptoms are evident. Restriction of protein and phosphorus with meticulous attention to blood pressure control may slow the course of progression.[69] At this time, evidence is lacking for instituting dietary modifications before symptoms are evident. However, there is good evidence that dietary counseling can be helpful once renal disease is symptomatic.

Residents with advanced renal insufficiency often suffer from anorexia, lassitude, and malnutrition, especially when weight loss is profound, uremic symptoms are evident, and dialysis is delayed. Anemia and osteoporosis are also common. Nutrition support of elderly residents with renal insufficiency is complex and demanding, since their metabolic derangements are not stable and vary over time as well as from one resident to another. Other diseases and conditions requiring diet therapy may also need attention.[70]

When GFR falls below 30 mL per minute, phosphate often accumulates and hyperphosphatemia results unless dietary phosphate is restricted. At the same time serum calcium concentration may decrease owing to increased serum phosphate, decreased production of $1,25(OH)_2D_3$ in the kidney, which leads to a decrease in calcium absorption from the gut and an impaired ability of parathyroid hormone to remove calcium from bone. Reduction in phosphorus intake from diet and the use of phosphate binders such as calcium carbonate at meals to bind with remaining phosphate in foods is often prescribed. Restriction of phosphorus levels to 600 to 900 mg per day can be achieved by decreasing the major dietary sources of phosphorus: milk and milk products, and meats. Currently calcium carbonate and other phosphate binders are preferred over aluminum salts because aluminum can be absorbed and may accumulate in body tissues.[71] These modifications help prevent the accumulation of phosphate in the blood, decrease parathyroid hormone levels, and improve its ability to remove calcium from bone if serum calcium levels fall too low.

However, the very foods that are restricted are also rich sources of calcium. For this reason calcium supplements of 500 to 1500 mg per day are needed to avoid negative calcium balance. The amounts vary, depending on the supplement used, the resident's size, serum calcium concentration, and other factors unique to the individual resident. In residents who are hypocalcemic and whose GFR is below 30 mL per minute, prescription of $1,25(OH)_2D_3$ also may be necessary to increase absorption. These dietary measures help keep plasma concentrations of calcium and phosphorus in normal ranges, prevent secondary hyperparathyroidism, and minimize risks of skeletal disease.

Residents who suffer from gastrointestinal conditions, such as peptic ulcer disease, often use large amounts of antacids and other over-the-counter medications without the knowledge of their physicians. If they are also being treated for advanced kidney disease, the use of over-the-counter medications may complicate therapy.[72]

Dialysis is life-saving for residents in chronic renal failure. However, it produces nutritional insults. Residents who are being dialyzed frequently appear cachexic and malnourished. The exact causes of the malnutrition vary from person to person, but include the catabolic nature of dialysis-induced alterations in nutrient metabolism, nutrient loss in the dialysate, and, frequently, intercurrent illness. Malnutrition is especially likely among residents who continue to have prolonged poor dietary intakes while they are being dialyzed. The nutritional depletion may contribute to the general debility and high morbidity from superimposed illnesses that are often present among such residents.[73]

In any event, the dietary objectives for renal patients are to ensure satisfactory quality of life while adjusting protein, potassium, sodium, and phosphorous intakes to maximize function.

Hepatic Disease

DEFINITION
Hepatic disease relates to diseases of the liver.

REASON FOR CONCERN
Aging has a major impact on both the anatomy and function of the liver. Liver size decreases; changes in many of its metabolic functions are apparent, including decreased rates of protein and enzyme synthesis, decreased induction of enzymes, decreased ability to metabolize toxic substances, and reduced gluconeogenetic activity.[74] The clinical problems resulting from these changes include increased risk of gallstones, altered metabolism of some drugs, and possible increased risk of some bacterial infections and immune disorders. Aging residents may require extra booster shots of some vaccines, such as hepatitis B. Also, alcohol may damage the sinusoidal cells of the liver more than it does in younger people.[75] The incidence of chronic, degenerative conditions affecting the liver (eg, gallbladder disease and cirrhosis) also rise with age. Current knowledge suggests that in health, the liver does not senesce as much as it withers. That is, its function is affected primarily by decreased activity of hepatocytes because of changes in extrahepatic hormones and mediators.

WELL-SUPPORTED INTERVENTIONS
Aging residents often suffer from diseases of the liver and biliary tract.[76] Hepatic encephalopathy may occur in acute liver failure due to several causes, such as alcoholism and viral hepatitis. Hepatic encephalopathy is due to extensive hepatic portal venous bypass and an excessive protein load. It is thought that the bacterial flora of the colon metabolize dietary amino acids to produce nitrogenous substances such as ammonia, bioactive amines

like tyramine and tryptamine, and mercaptans, which all may have cerebrotoxic effects. These substances are absorbed, and when a portacaval shunt is present, the blood supply bypasses the liver, where nitrogenous substances normally are cleared from the blood and detoxified, and reaches the brain directly. The hyperammonemia is closely associated with the development of episodes of tremor, which can progress to delirium and coma.

The dietary therapy of advanced liver disease is complex. If the resident is malnourished, rehabilitation is important. For alcoholic liver disease without cirrhosis, or for other liver disease, nutrition therapy often results in clinical improvement and better quality of life. Energy intake should be high, and carbohydrate intake should be high enough to prevent catabolism of body tissue. Protein intake should be sufficient to meet needs for rehabilitation, and minerals and vitamins should equal or exceed RDA levels. Residents with liver disease are often anorectic and so ill that special enteral feedings must be employed. There is good evidence that nutritional status can be improved by nutrition support, but whether morbidity and mortality rates change as well is still unclear.[77,78]

In advanced liver disease, it is important to ensure that intakes of vitamins are adequate. Disordered secretion of bile may inhibit absorption of the fat-soluble vitamins. Other vitamins that are extensively metabolized in the liver, such as vitamin K or folacin, also need to be provided in supplement form.

When advanced liver disease is complicated by hepatic encephalopathy, the situation is more complicated. Residents with cirrhosis and evidence of protein-energy malnutrition need special care, since they have low tolerance of high-protein diets, and the need to avoid precipitating hepatic encephalopathy is an important consideration. Even intakes of protein approximating the RDA may precipitate hepatic encephalopathy. Thus, current theory is to maintain protein at 20 to 30 g per day to keep mentation satisfactory. But at these levels of intake, protein-energy malnutrition is likely. Some experts who agree with the amino acid imbalance theory use enteral or parenteral feedings of low aromatic amino acid and high branched chain amino acid at 60 to 80 g per day. Intakes of these mixtures appear to improve nitrogen balance, but may not eliminate hepatic encephalopathy.[79]

Immune System Disease

DEFINITION

The two major categories of immune deficiency disorders are primary and secondary disorders.[80] The primary immune deficiency disorders are diseases in and of themselves. All are rare, involving heredity or acquired defects of B or T lymphocytes, phagocytes, or complement; more than half the cases are due to antibody-mediated immune disorders of the B lymphocytes. All cause their victims to suffer recurring infections.

Secondary immune deficiency disorders are the result of other diseases.

The disordered immune system then causes further complications. The most common cause of secondary immune disorders are chemotherapeutic and other agents that suppress the bone marrow and alter T and B lymphocyte production. Immunosuppression during transplants is also essential to avoid organ rejection. Secondary immune deficiency is involved in illnesses like leukemia, in which malignant cells replace normal populations of T or B lymphocytes. Bacterial infections causing sepsis overwhelm the immune system and cause secondary immune deficiency. Finally, there is acquired immunodeficiency syndrome (AIDS) caused by human immunodeficiency virus (HIV) infection.

REASON FOR CONCERN

Immune competence declines with age; for example, T lymphocyte function decreases. It is not known whether these changes, sometimes referred to as *immunosenescence*, are inevitable consequences of aging. Current thinking is that while some of the changes may be inevitable, many due to disease are preventable or treatable. Many autoimmune diseases and therapies that alter immune response have nutritional implications. Malnutrition may also worsen disease-caused weakening of the immune system, thus increasing susceptibility to infection.

The widespread hypothesis that compromised immune status in elderly residents results from malnutrition, often brings residents to ask what they can eat to improve immune function.[81] Therefore, it is important for health professionals to be well informed about the links between nutrition, immune function, and aging.

WELL-SUPPORTED INTERVENTIONS

The popular theory that immunosenescence is due to malnutrition has not been borne out by research studies.[82]

Severe protein-energy malnutrition does alter the proportion of T-cell types, depresses T-cell function, and impairs both delayed hypersensitivity and thymic factor activity, and these changes may increase susceptibility to infectious diseases. Among those who are severely malnourished and suffer from protein-energy malnutrition due to inadequate dietary intake, some— but not all—of their immune function defects are reversed by nutrition support. Immunocompetence is not restored by nutrition support in those who are severely malnourished with wasting diseases such as cancer or HIV infection that alter immune function.

Specific nutrient deficiencies, such as zinc deficiency, alter some tests of immune function.[83] However, zinc supplementation has variable and not always positive effects in improving antibody responses.[84,85]

Some studies report that dietary supplements of vitamins, minerals, or other nutrients improve antibody responses to viral vaccines among older people. It is unclear if these effects are due to supplements or to simultaneous treatment of underlying illnesses.[86,87]

Some elderly residents are immunosuppressed as side effects of treatment for organ or marrow transplants and immunosuppressive chemotherapy given for certain cancers, severe arthritis, early primary biliary cirrhosis, and other diseases. After a course of immunosuppressive therapy they may be debilitated and in need of nutrition support to restore lost weight and lean body mass.

Diseases such as HIV infection cause immunosuppression. When HIV infection is present, the goals of dietary treatment are to preserve lean body mass and to prevent dietary deficiencies, including protein-energy malnutrition and vitamin and mineral deficiencies.[88] Special dietary modifications may be needed to provide symptomatic relief for the many opportunistic infections that arise.

Other diseases common among the elderly alter some aspects of immune function, although they do not suppress it. Examples include severe liver disease. The diet therapy of liver disease is discussed earlier in this chapter.

Rheumatoid arthritis and some other autoimmune diseases of elderly people have nutritional implications. Nutrition neither causes nor cures rheumatoid arthritis or osteoarthritis (which is not an autoimmune disease). Arthritis victims need to avoid the questionable dietary remedies that abound for treating the condition; some are dangerous, and there is little evidence to support their claims.[89] Elderly residents who have osteoarthritis of weight-bearing joints sometimes experience symptomatic relief from weight reduction if they are obese. It is easier to walk and perform daily activities when they carry less weight.

Sjögren's syndrome is an autoimmune disease that causes decreased saliva production, dry mouth, and, consequently, difficulties in eating and rampant dental caries. It is treated by alterations in dietary consistency, consumption of noncariogenic foods, and scrupulous oral hygiene.

Dementia (Especially Alzheimer's Disease)

DEFINITION

Dementia is a syndrome that involves decreased mental performance, particularly loss of many aspects of language, learning, memory, thinking, and reasoning. Both temporary and permanent causes of dementia occur in the elderly.

The major causes of dementia in older residents are senile dementia of the Alzheimer's type (SDAT), multi-infarct dementia (MID), drug- and alcohol-related dementias, and those due to other, less age-specific causes. Diet may be involved in the causation of dementias due to dehydration and vitamin B_{12} deficiency due to pernicious anemia.

REASON FOR CONCERN

Most mental functions decline as a result of diseases and conditions that accompany aging, and are not inevitable, age-associated events.[90]

Among the most formidable of the challenges facing nutrition professionals is the nutrition care of elderly residents who suffer from Alzheimer's disease and related disorders. Alzheimer's disease is a progressive brain disorder marked by the slow deterioration of the mind. At present, ways to prevent or cure the disease are unknown. It afflicts more than 2 million middle-aged and older adults. The incidence of Alzheimer's disease rises sharply with age. While only between 5% and 8% of all those aged 65 and over are affected, the incidence in the population older than age 85 is 35%.[91] The costs of caring for those who are afflicted are very high—between $30 billion and $80 billion—because eventually most residents are institutionalized.[92] In the next 50 years, as more and more Americans reach the eighth and ninth decades of life, the incidence can be expected to triple.

Multi-infarct dementia, another common cause of dementia in elderly residents, results from arteriosclerotic disease. Its causes and prevention are better understood, but because cardiovascular and arteriosclerotic disease are so common in the elderly, its incidence and prevalence are also likely to remain high for the foreseeable future.

Dehydration is a common cause of lethargy, lightheadedness, altered mental status, confusional states, and dementia in elderly residents. Older adults have lower body water content and an impaired sense of thirst, their kidneys cannot concentrate a solute load to the same extent, and they take more diuretics than younger people.

Drug-induced dementias are common in elderly residents because so many are medicated and adverse reactions to drugs are more common. More than half of all older people take at least one medication daily, and many take multiple drugs.[93]

The elderly also suffer from both permanent and transient dementias resulting from many other causes that are not as highly associated with age: untreated pernicious anemia, infections, complications of diabetes mellitus, heart disease, pulmonary disease, depression, alcohol abuse, and some forms of malnutrition such as protein-energy malnutrition also increase risks of malnutrition.

WELL-SUPPORTED INTERVENTIONS.

The causes of Alzheimer's disease are obscure. Age, family history of Alzheimer's disease, and head injuries increase risk. Nutritional risk factors are not thought to play a role. The brain lesions that are characteristic of Alzheimer's disease contain aluminum. Originally it was thought that high aluminum intake causes the disease. However, there is little evidence that renal dialysis or the use of aluminum antacids, antiperspirants, or aluminum cookware increases Alzheimer's disease risk.[94] Also, some people who die of other causes and exhibited no signs of Alzheimer's disease also have high aluminum concentrations in the neurons of their brains.[95] The possibility that lecithin or choline in the diet might restore levels of acetylcholine in the brain to normal levels in Alzheimer's disease was tested a decade ago and failed.

Alzheimer's residents do best in a simple, highly structured environment with regular meals. Residents often become confused, so menu item choices should be kept simple. Food should be served at eating temperatures since the person may lack the judgment to wait until very hot foods cool. They need greater mealtime supervision than do other residents.

Judgment, memory, and coordination deteriorate as the disease progresses, making eating more difficult. Finger foods like sandwiches and burgers, are easy to eat. Some spilling is inevitable, and clothing worn at mealtime should be washable. Feeding an SDAT resident is not the same as feeding a young baby or child. The differences are not always obvious unless they are pointed out and proper techniques demonstrated. To identify problems, the registered dietitian must observe SDAT residents while they eat. Appropriate feeding techniques help minimize risks of aspiration. Demented residents who refuse to eat and make strange mouth movements may have dental problems or ill-fitting dentures. Regular dental checkups can help to prevent this.

In the later stages of Alzheimer's disease, eating becomes increasingly difficult, and the resident may have to be fed. Lack of appetite and forgetting to eat to the point where emaciation is the result are risks. Alzheimer's disease and some of the other dementias involve progressive cognitive and functional deterioration.[96] Nutritional status often deteriorates as mental and physical capabilities decline. Residents are confused and easily distracted, and in the late stages may require feeding assistance or enteral feedings to meet energy needs. They are unable to communicate their malaise if they are ill, so that without very careful surveillance, illnesses and fever may go undetected. For example, in one recent study intakes of energy and nutrients were lower than two thirds of the RDAs among nursing facility residents with SDAT than among controls. The energy output of SDAT residents who were "wanderers" was high, but not always compensated for by increased intakes.[97]

Even when their energy intakes are seemingly adequate, SDAT residents are often undernourished and underweight. In part this may be due to the presence of occult infections that go undetected, such as those of the urinary tract.[98] Another explanation is the extreme difficulty involved in feeding very deteriorated residents who are unable to eat by themselves. In another study, SDAT residents entered a nursing facility underweight and continued to lose weight in the next year and a half, presumably because of feeding management issues.[99] The possibility that there are metabolic aberrations inherent in the disease itself has also been raised, but never demonstrated.

Once feeding assistance is needed, the time and patience it requires may exceed the ability of the caregiver. In nursing facilities, several different staff members usually are involved in assisting a given resident. They may be unaware of what the other staff members are doing or of what the resident has eaten during the rest of the day. While they may be kind and well meaning, they often lack the determination to ensure that intakes are adequate. The potential for elder abuse is present both in home and institutional settings; signs of abuse must be investigated especially when the resident appears to be fearful or frightened. Adequate staffing, training, and supervision of caregivers and routine monitoring of food intake and weight on an ongoing basis prevent unnecessary deterioration in nutritional status. All caregivers who feed residents need patience and training.

Multi-infarct dementias due to arteriosclerosis of the blood vessels of the brain can cause permanent dementias involving cognitive losses, depression, and other behavior changes. Hemorrhagic stroke caused by rupture of cerebral blood vessels and occlusive stroke caused by atherosclerosis both increase with age. Stroke often causes partial paralysis, aphasia, and depressive emotional changes. In addition, chewing and swallowing often are affected, making alimentation difficult and increasing risks of aspiration. While some improvements usually occur in the first year after a stroke, some are permanent. Assistive feeding devices, modifications in food texture, and use of liquid nutritional supplements can help ensure adequate alimentation. If the gag reflex is absent, or if the resident constantly aspirates food or fluids, use of other nutrition support systems should be considered.

Residents who have experienced occlusive strokes are often placed on the anticoagulant warfarin (Coumadin*) preventively. Warfarin is an antagonist to vitamin K, and supplements or foods very high in vitamin K should be avoided. Warfarin's action is affected by sudden changes in alcohol and food intake. Other types of cardiovascular and pulmonary disease sometimes cause anoxia of brain tissues and temporary dementia that is often reversible with medication or other treatment. Severe heart disease, high blood pressure, and arrhythmias are other common vascular problems among the elderly that affect memory and learning. Frail, demented elderly residents often eat improperly and become malnourished unless help is provided.

Dehydration is preventable by ensuring that the elderly drink fluids frequently. Planning meals that include adequate fluids, keeping diuretic medications properly adjusted, and making special efforts to ensure hydration during periods of heat stress, fever, diarrhea, vomiting, and ketoacidosis may keep the resident hydrated. A good target to aim for is 1.5 to 2 L of fluid per day, especially if the resident is on a high-fiber diet. Nocturnal dehydration and dehydration during illness should be avoided by putting water pitchers within reach of the bed and counseling the resident and staff about the importance of fluid intake. Fever and infection are other reversible causes of dementia, particularly if accompanied by dehydration. The underlying problem can be treated with medicine and nutritional measures that ensure hydration.

---

* DuPont Pharmaceuticals, Wilmington, DE 19880.

Drug-related problems are preventable causes of dementia in elderly residents. Some of the more common drugs causing cognitive impairment in the elderly are diuretics, digitalis, barbiturates, thyroid preparations in the wrong doses, and mixtures of antidepressants and alcohol. Some drugs affect appetite. Drugs that stimulate appetite include some of the phenothiazines such as chlorpromazine (Thorazine*) or epinephrine and the opioid peptides. Drugs that cause anorexia include dopamine, epinephrine, serotonin, amphetamines, and high doses of antidepressants such as fluoxetine (Prozac†).[100] Fortunately other drugs are available that do not produce these side effects. The registered dietitian can help by pointing out any obvious drug-nutrient or drug-drug combinations that are affecting the resident.

Drunkenness is a cause of acute and transient periods of confusion, memory problems, and even delirium. Elderly people have lower tolerance for alcohol and are particularly prone to those problems. Chronic alcoholism coupled with years of malnutrition increase risks of Korsakoff's encephalopathy, or the Wernicke-Korsakoff syndrome: loss of recent memory, intellectual loss, and gait disorders. Because of memory problems most of these residents must be institutionalized.

The treatment of dementia often employs antipsychotic medications to control disturbing behaviors like severe agitation, violence, and paranoia. Some drugs have anorectic or orexigenic (appetite-stimulating) properties. Long, continued use of certain antipsychotic medications sometimes leads to tardive dyskinesia, which involves uncontrolled and exaggerated movements of the mouth, tongue, and jaw area. The best way to control this is to avoid or discontinue any drug that causes it, and to regulate medications precisely.

Undiagnosed vitamin B_{12} deficiency is also a cause of dementia. Sometimes serum B_{12} levels decline as residents age.[101] Although the incidence of atrophic gastritis with consequent reduction in gastric acid production and stomach acidity occurs, the use of B_{12} increases risks of bacterial overgrowth. The major causes of these decreased levels are usually not diet-related, except in elderly residents who have eaten no animal foods for many years and who refuse vitamin supplements. Vitamin B_{12} malabsorption due to the increased prevalence of pernicious anemia and atrophic gastritis coupled with bacterial overgrowth rises with age.[102] Pernicious anemia is due to lack of intrinsic factor secretion by the gastric mucosa and is especially prevalent with aging in northern Europeans and American blacks. It is thought to be due to an autoimmune reaction against gastric parietal cells causing gastric atrophy. A characteristic macrocytic anemia then develops. However, even in residents with normal blood pictures neurologic disease may occur. Confusion and mental changes are among the earliest signs of vitamin B_{12} deficiency. They vary from mild irritability to forgetfulness, psychosis, and frank dementia. If identified and treated

---

* SmithKline Beecham Pharmaceuticals, Philadelphia, PA 19101.
† Dista Products Co, Div of Eli Lilly and Co, Indianapolis, IN 46285.

early, the symptoms are reversible. When they continue undetected, demyelination progresses, axonal degeneration and eventual neuronal death occurs. If symptoms do not remit on treatment, brain function may be permanently damaged.[103]

Summary

The nutrition needs of the healthy elderly are similar but not the same as those of their younger peers and are further altered by the various diseases and conditions from which they frequently suffer.[104] The nutritional status of the elderly are affected by disease, poor food intake, and frailty. The assessment of the nutritional status of older residents should include anthropometric measurements, biochemical indexes, clinical examination and history, and dietary intake data.[105] Functional status, including the activities of daily living and instrumental activities of daily living, also must be determined since it explains differences in quality of life that are not described by diagnoses alone.[106] Above all, dietary therapy must be approached with common sense, a flexible and liberal attitude, and respect for residents' dietary preferences. This will maximize the probability of a better quality of life for their remaining years.

References

1.   Dean W. Biological age. In: Anacker PC, Kaufman RC, Weber HU, eds. *Biological Aging Measurement: Clinical Applications*. 2nd ed. Los Angeles, Calif: Center for Bio Gerontology; 1988:3–20.
2.   Borkan GA. Factors in clinical aging: variation in rates of aging. In: Regelson W, Sinex FM, eds. *Intervention in the Aging Process Part A. Quantitation, Epidemiology, and Clinical Research*. New York, NY: Alan R Liss Inc; 1983:99–112.
3.   Regelson W. Biomarkers and aging. In: Regelson W, Sinex FM, eds. *Intervention in the Aging Process Part A. Quanitation, Epidemiology, and Clinical Research*. New York, NY: Alan R Liss Inc; 1983:3–98.
4.   Metropolitan Life Insurance Company. Tables of desirable weight for height. *Metropolitan Life Insurance Company Statistical Bulletin*. 1983.
5.   Frisancho AR. New Standards of weight and body composition by frame size and height for assessment of nutritional status of adults and the elderly. *Am J Clin Nutr.* 1984;40:808–819.
6.   Shuman CR. Optimum insulin use in older diabetics. *Geriatrics* 1984; 39:71.
7.   Reaven GM, Reaven EP. Age, glucose intolerance, and non-insulin-dependent diabetes mellitus. J Am Geriatrics Soc. 1985;33:286–290.
8.   Kahn SE, Schwartz RS, Porte D, et al. The glucose intolerance of aging: implications for intervention. *Hosp Pract*. 1991;1:29–38.
9.   Subcommittee on Hypertension Definition and Prevalence, Joint, National Committee on the Detection, Evaluation, and Treatment of High Blood Pressure. Hypertension prevalence and the status of awareness, treatment and control in the United States. *Hypertension*. 1985;7:457–465.
10.   Lakatta EG. Mechanisms of hypertension in the elderly. *J Am Geriatr Soc*. 1980;37:780–790.
11.   Williamson J, Chapin JM. Adverse reactions to prescribed drugs in the elderly: a multicenter investigation. *Aging*. 1980;9:73–80.

12. Knapp HR. Hypertension. In: Brown ML, ed. *Present Knowledge in Nutrition.* 6th ed. Washington, DC: International Life Sciences Institute-Nutrition Foundation; 1990:355-361.

13. Abbott RD, Garrision RJ, Wilson PWF, et al. Joint distribution of lipoprotein cholesterol classes: the Framingham study. *Arteriosclerosis.* 1983;3:260-272.

14. Ericsson S, Eriksson M, Vitols S, Einarsson K, Berglund L, Angeline B. Influence of age on the metabolism of plasma low density lipoproteins in healthy males. *J Clin Invest.* 1991;87:591-596.

15. Grundy SM, Vega GL, Bilheimer DW. Kinetic mechanisms determining variability in low density lipoprotein levels and rises with age. *Arteriosclerosis.* 1985;5:623-630.

16. Heart disease. In: *The Surgeon General's Report on Nutrition and Health.* Washington DC: Dept of Health and Human Services. Public Health Service, US Government Printing Office; 1988. DHHS (PHS) publication 88-50210.

17. Sytkowski PA, Kannel WB, Agosinao RB. Changes in risk factors and the decline in mortality from cardiovascular disease: the Framingham heart study. *N Engl J Med.* 1990;322:1635-1640.

18. Gordon T, Rifkind B. Treating high blood cholesterol in the older patient. *Am J Cardiol.* 1989;63:48H-52H.

19. Garn SN, Rohmann CG, Nolan P. The developmental nature of bone changes during aging. In: Burren JE, ed. *Relations of Development and Aging.* Springfield, Ill: Charles C Thomas; 1980:41-61.

20. Kraenzlin ME, Jennings JC, Baylink DJ. Calcium and bone homeostasis with aging. In: Andres R, Bierman EL, Hazzard WR, eds. *Principles of Geriatric Medicine.* 2nd ed. New York, NY: McGraw Hill; 1985:799-812.

21. National Institute of Arthritis, Musculoskeletal, and Skin Diseases, *Osteoporosis: Cause, Treatment and Prevention.* Bethesda, Md: National Institutes of Health; 1984. NIH publication 86-2226.

22. Krall EA, Sayhoun N, Tannenbaum S, Dallal GE, Dawson HB. Effect of vitamin D intake on seasonal variations in parathyroid hormone secretion in postmenopausal women. *N Engl J Med* 1989;321:1777-1783.

23. Chestnut CH. Ostoporosis. In: Jandres R, Bierman EL, Hazzard WL. *Principles of Geriatric Medicine and Gerontology.* 2nd ed. New York, NY: McGraw Hill; 1985:813-325.

24. Riggs BL, Melton LJ. Medical progress: involutional osteoporosis. *N Engl J Med.* 1986;314:1676-1684.

25. Bastow MD, Rifking J, Alison SR. Benefits of supplementary tube feeding after fractured neck of femus: a randomised controlled trial. *Br Med J.* 1983;287:1589-1592.

26. Delmi M, Rapin CH, Bengoa JM, Delmas PD, Vasey H, Bonjour JP. Dietary supplementation in elderly patients with fractured neck of the femus. *Lancet* 1990;1:1013-1016.

27. Brody JA, Brock DB, Williams TF. Trends in the health of the elderly population. *Annu Rev Public Health.* 1987;8:211-234.

28. Donahoe M, Rogers RM, Wilson DO, Pennock BE. Oxygen consumption of the respiratory muscles in normal and malnourished patients with chronic obstructive pulmonary disease. *Am Rev Respir Dis.* 1989;140:385-391.

29. Terry PB. Chronic airways obstruction and respiratory failure. In: Andres R, Bierman EL, Hazzard WR, eds. *Principles of Geriatric Medicine.* 2nd ed. New York, NY: McGraw Hill;1985:526-537.

30. Mohsensin V, Feranti R, Like JS, et al. Nutrition for the respiratory insufficient patient. *Eur Respir J.* 1989;2:663a-665b.

31. Fiaccadori E, Del Dnale S, Coffrini E, et al. Hypercapnic-hypoxemic chronic obstructive pulmonary disease (COPD): influence of severity of COPD on nutritional status. *Am J Clin Nutr.* 1988;48:680-685.

32. Lewis MI, Belman MJ, Dorr Uyemura L. Nutrition and the respiratory muscles. *Clin Chest Med.* 1988;9:337-348.

33. Wilson DO, Donahoe M, Rogers RM, Pennock BE. Metabolic rate and weight loss in chronic obstructive lung disease. *JPEN J Parenter Enteral Nutr.* 1990;14:7-11.

34. Donahoe M, Rogers RM, Wilson DO. Oxygen consumption of the respiratory muscles in normal and in malnourished patient with chronic obstructive pulmonary disease. *Am Rev Respir Dis.* 1989;140:385-391.

35. Donahoe M, Rogers RM. Nutritional assessment and support in chronic obstructive pulmonary disease. *Clin Chest Med.* 1990;11:487-504.

36. Keim NL, Luby MH, Braun SR, Martin AM, Dixon RM. Dietary evaluation of outpatients with chronic obstructive pulmonary disease. *J Am Diet Assoc.* 1986;86:902-906.

37. Barrocas A, Tretola R, Alonso A. Nutrition and the critically ill pulmonary patient. *Resp Care.* 1983;28:50-59.

38. Edelman NH, Rucker RB, Peavy HH. NIH workshop summary: nutrition and the respiratory system. Chronic obstructive pulmonary disease (COPD). *Am Rev Respir Dis.* 1986;134:347-352.

39. Goldstein S, Askanazi J, Weissman C, Thomashow B, Kenney JM. Energy expenditure in patients with chronic obstructive pulmonary disease. *Chest.* 1987;91:222-224.

40. Geulpa G, Chevrolet JC. Nonspecific chronic obstructive bronchopneumopathy and nutrition. *Schweiz Med Wochenschr.* 1978;117:168-172.

41. Openbrier DR, Covey M. Ineffective breathing pattern related to malnutrition. *Nurs Clin North Am.* 1987;22:225-247.

42. Tockman MS. Aging of the respiratory system. In: Andres R, Bierman EL, Hazzard WL, eds. *Principles of Geriatric Medicine and Gerontology.* 2nd ed. New York, NY: McGraw Hill; 1985:499-507.

43. Efthimiou J, Fleming J, Gomes C, Spiro SG. The effect of supplmentary oral nutrition in poorly nourished patients with chronic obstructive pulmonary disease. *Am Rev Respir Dis.* 1988;137:1075-1082.

44. Knowles JB, Firbarn MS, Wiggs BJ, Chan Yan C, Pardy RL. Dietary supplementation and respiratory muscle performance in patients with COPD. *Chest.* 1988;93:977-983.

45. Hodgkin JE. Prognosis in chronic obstructive pulmonary disease. *Clin Chest Med.* 1990;11:555-569.

46. Goldstein SA, Thomashow B, Askanazi J. Functional changes during nutritional repletion in patients with lung disease. *Clin Chest Med.* 1986;7:141-151.

47. Kritchevsky D. Cancer. In: Brown M, ed. *Present Knowledge in Nutrition.* 6th ed. Washington, DC: International Life Sciences Institute–Nutrition Foundation; 1990:395-398.

48. *Cancer Statistics 1990.* New York, NY: American Cancer Society; 1990.

49. Moldower LL, Lowry SF, Cerami A. Cachectin. Its impact on metabolism and nutritional status. *Annu Rev Nutr.* 1988;8:585-609.

50. Nixon DW, Heymsfield SB, Cohen AB, et al. Protein calorie undernutrition in hospitalized cancer patients. *Am J Med.* 1980;68:683-690.

51. Dwyer JT. Nutrition education of the cancer patient and family: myths and realities. *Cancer.* 1986;58:1887-1896.

52. *Unconventional Cancer Treatments.* Washington, DC: Office of Technology Assessment, US Congress, US Government Printing Office; 1990.

53. *Quackery and the Elderly.* New York, NY: American Council on Science and Health; 1990.

54. Chapman N, Sorenson A, Ory MG, Monjan A. Nature, causes and consequences of harmful dietary practices: implications for older people. *Clin Appl Nutr.* 1991;1:32-51.

55. Shils ME. Nutrition and diet in cancer. In: Shils ME, Young VR. *Modern Nutrition in Health and Disease.* 7th ed. Philadelphia, Pa: Lea & Febiger; 1988:1380–1422.

56. American Cancer Society. *Second National Conference on Diet, Nutrition and Cancer* 1986;58(suppl):1791–1962.

57. Nutritional management of the cancer patient. In: *Manual of Clinical Dietetics.* Chicago, Ill: The American Dietetic Association; 1989:301–305.

58. Smith TJ, Dwyer JT, La Francesca JP. Nutrition and the cancer patient. In: Osteen RT, ed. *Cancer Manual.* 8th ed. Boston, Mass: American Cancer Society, Massachusetts Division; 1990:498.

59. Dwyer JT, Roy J. Diet therapy. In: Wilson JD, Braunwald E, Isselbacher KJ, et al, eds. *Harrison's Principles of Internal Medicine.* 12th ed. New York, NY: McGraw Hill; 1990:420–427.

60. Szeluga DJ, et al. Nutritional support of bone marrow transplant recipients: a prospective randomized clinical trial comparing total parenteral nutrition to an enteral feeding program. *Cancer Res.* 1987;47:3309.

61. Weisdorf S, et al. Influence of prophylactic total parenteral nutrition on long term outcome of bone marrow transplantation. *Transplant.* 1987;43:833.

62. Howard L. Parenteral and enteral nutrition therapy. In: Wilson JD, Braunwald EP, Isselbacher K, et al, eds. *Harrison's Principles of Internal Medicine.* 12th ed. New York: NY. McGraw Hill; 1990:427–434.

63. Dwyer JT. The spectrum of dietary and nutritional approaches to cancer. *Nutr Rep.* 1989;4:197–199.

64. American Society for Parenteral and Enteral Nutrition. Guidelines. *JPEN J Parenter Enteral Nutr.* 1986;10:441; 1987;11:342,439.

65. Howard L. Parenteral and enteral nutrition. In: Wilson JD, Braunwald E, Isselbacher KJ, et al, eds. *Harrison's Principles of Internal Medicine.* 12th ed. New York, NY: McGraw Hill; 1990:75.

66. Theologides A. Nutritional management of the patient with advanced cancer. *Postgrad Med.* 1977;61:97–101.

67. Gallagher-Allred CR. *Nutritional Care of the Terminally Ill.* Gaithersburg, Md: Aspen Publishers; 1989.

68. Meyer BR. Renal function in aging. *J Am Geriatr Soc.* 1989;37:791–860.

69. Ihle BU, Becker GT, Whitworth JA, Charlwood RA, Kincaid-Smith PS. The effect of protein restriction on the progressional of renal insuffiency. *N Engl J Med* 1989;321:1773–1777.

70. Shapiro E, Carbry J, Stollar C, Dwyer JT. Renal diet exchange lists: evaluation of potential teachability and precision. *Top Clin Nutr.* 1991;7:63–71.

71. Slatopolsky E, Weerts C, Lopez-Hilker S, et al. Calcium carbonate as a phosphate binder in patients with chronic renal failure undergoing dialysis. *N Engl J Med.* 1986;315:157–161.

72. Shikora SA, Driscoll DF, Bistrian BR. Metabolic alkalosis in a patient with renal failure: role of antacids. *Nutr Rev.* 1990;48:2147–2150.

73. Feinstein E, Massry S. Nutritonal therapy in acute renal failure. In: Mitch WE, Klahr S, eds. *Nutrition and the Kidney.* Boston, Mass: Little Brown and Co; 1988;80–103.

74. Shephard RJ. Nutrition and the physiology of aging. In: Young EA, ed. *Nutrition, Aging and Health.* New York, NY: Alan R Liss Inc; 1985:1–23.

75. Popper H. Hepatic problems in aging. In: Bianchi L, Holt P, James OFW, Butler RN. *Aging in the Liver and Gastrointestinal Tract.* Lancaster, England: MTP Press Ltd; 1987:383–388.

76. Strom BL, West SL. The epidemiology of gallstone disease. In: Cohen S, Soloway RD, eds. *Contemporary Issues in Gastroenterology.* New York, NY: Churchill Livingstone; 1985:1–26.

77. Achord JL. A randomized controlled trial of peripheral amino acid glucose infusion in acute alcoholic hepatitis. *Am J Gastroenterol.* 1987;82:871–875a.

78. Calvey H, Davis M, Williams R. Controlled trial of nutritional supplementation with and without branched amino acid enrichment in the treatment of acute alcoholic hepatitis. *J Hepatol.* 1985;1:141–151.

79. Alexander WF, Spindel E, Harty RF, Cerda JJ. The usefulness of branched chain amino acids in patients with acute or chronic hepatic encephalopathy. Am J Gastroenterol. 1989;84:91–96.

80. Benjamini E, Leskowitz S. *Immunology: A Short Course.* 2nd ed. New York, NY: Wiley Liss; 211–233.

81. Thompson JS, Robbins J, Cooper JK. Nutrition and immune function in the geriatric population. *Clin Geriatric Med.* 1987;3:309–317.

82. Shock NW, Gruelich RC, Costa PT, et al. *Human Aging: the Baltimore Longitudinal Study of Aging.* Bethesda, Md: US Dept of Agriculture National Institute of Health; 1984:137–147. USDA/NIH publication 84-2450.

83. Gershwin ME, Beach R, Hurley L. Trace metals, aging, and immunity. *J Am Geriatr Soc.* 1983;31:374–378.

84. Duchateau J, Delespesse G, Virjens R, Collet H. Beneficial effects of oral zinc supplementation on the immune response of old people. *Am J Med.* 1981;70:1001–1004.

85. Brader MD, Hollingsworth JW, Saltner PD, Strause LG, Klauber MR, Lugo NJ. Failure of oral zinc supplementation to improve the antibody response to influenza vaccine. *Nutr Res.* 1988;8:99-104.

86. Chandra RK, Puri S. Nutritional support improves antibody response to influenza virus vaccine in the elderly. *Br Med J.* 1985;291:705-706.

87. Goodwin JS, Garry PJ. Relationship between megadose vitamin supplementation and immunological function in a healthy elderly population. *Clin Exper Immunol.* 1983;51:647–653.

88. Dwyer JT. Nutrition support of HIV+ patients. *Henry Ford Hospital Med J.* 1991;39:60–65.

89. Dwyer JT. Questionable dietary therapies in immunology. In: Klurfeld D, ed. *Nutrition and Immunology.* In press.

90. Palmore E. Mental aging. In: *Normal Aging. Reports from the Duke Longitudinal Studies. 1970–1973.* Durham, NC: Duke University Press; 1974;12:87–150.

91. US Department of Health and Human Services. Aging. In: *The Surgeon General's Report on Nutrition and Health.* Washington, DC: US Government Printing Office; 1988: 595-627. DHHS publication (PHS) 88-50210.

92. Huange LS, Cartwright WS, Hu TW. Economic cost of senile dementia. In: *US Pub Health Rep.* 1985;103:3-7.

93. Lecos CW. Diet and the elderly: watch out for food drug mismatches. *FDA Consumer.* 1984-1985;18:7–9.

94. Katzman R. Alzheimer's disease. *N Engl J Med.* 1986;314:964–973.

95. Perl DP, Brody AR. Alzheimer's disease: x-ray spectrometric evidence of aluminum accumulation in neurofibrally tangle bearing neurons. *Science* 1980;208:297-299.

96. Pearson JL, Teri L, Reifler BV, Raskind MA. Functional status and cognitive impairment in Alzheimer's patients with and without depression. *J Am Geriatr Soc.* 1989;37:1117-1121.

97. Litchford MD, Wakefield LM. Nutrient intakes and energy expenditures of residents with senile dementia of the Alzheimer's type. *J Am Diet Assoc.* 1987;87:211-213.

98. Sandman PO, Adolfsson R, Nygren C, et al. Nutritional status and dietary intake in institutionalized patients with Alzheimer's disease and multiinfarct dementia. *J Am Gerontol Soc.* 1987;35:31–38.

99. Franklin CA, Karkeck J. Weight loss and senile dementia in an institutionalized elderly population. *J Am Diet Assoc.* 1989;89:790–792.

100. Sullivan AC, Gruen RK. Mechanisms of appetite modulation by drugs. *Fed Proc.* 1985;44:129–144.

101.   Elsborg I, Lund V, Bastrup-Madsen P. Serum vitamin B_{12} levels in the aged. *Acta Med Scand.* 1976;200:309–314.

102.   Suter PM, Russell RM. Vitamin requirements of the elderly. *Am J Clin Nutr.* 1987;45:501–512.

103.   Babior BM, Bunn HF. Megaloblastic anemias. In: Wilson JD, Braunwald E, Isselbacher KJ, et al, eds. *Harrison's Principles of Internal Medicine.* 12th ed. New York, NY: McGraw Hill; 1991:523–529.

104.   Blumberg JB. Considerations of the Recommended Dietary Allowances for older adults. *Clin Appl Nutr.* 1991;11:9–18.

105.   Mitchell CO. Nutritional assessment of the elderly. *Clin Appl Nutr.* 1991;1:76–88.

106.   Dwyer J, Coletti J, Campbell D. Maximizing nutrition in the second fifty. *Clin Appl Nutr.* 1991;1:19–32.

3. Risk Factors Associated With Poor Nutritional Status

Risk Factor Definition

Nutritional Risk Factors

Selected Acute and Chronic Diseases or Conditions

3. RISK FACTORS ASSOCIATED WITH POOR NUTRITIONAL STATUS

Aging is a complex process. Its dimensions are defined by the interplay of complex and diverse life events experienced over time. Because genetic makeup and human response are unique to each person, the process of aging is characterized by heterogeneity.[1] Nutrition needs and concerns in older people tend to be multifactorial and are not always easy to identify or meet.[2,3] While it is apparent that physiologic systems wear out at different rates, it remains unclear how much of this variability is generic to the aging process, and how much is due to failure to change attitudes and behaviors that negatively impact health.[1,4-6]

This chapter will discuss risk factors associated with poor nutritional status in older persons. Definitions of the risk factors will be provided, reasons for concern will be identified, and general recommendations regarding appropriate intervention will be described.

Although this publication is directed primarily to nursing facility providers, parts of this chapter deal with a variety of economic and social factors. While these factors may not always be perceived as applicable to the nursing home resident of long duration, they are extremely relevant to admission and discharge planning. Residents frequently leave the nursing facility for periods to be admitted to acute care facilities, or rehabilitative centers, or to return home. The economic and social factors described are relevant to these situations.

Providers must remember that it is important to view each older adult as a unique person with specific needs. Individualized nutrition care plans that are designed to accommodate specific identified needs are the hallmark of quality nutrition care.

Risk Factor Definition

A *risk factor* is a characteristic or occurrence that increases the likelihood that a person will have a nutrition problem(s).[7] Obviously, the greater the number of these occurrences or characteristics an individual experiences, and the longer they persist, the greater the likelihood of poor nutritional status.

Nutritional Risk Factors

A variety of medical and psychosocial stressors have the potential to impact nutritional status negatively. Recognition of their presence often serves as an "early warning sign" of impending malnutrition. Many causes of poor nutritional status can be anticipated and prevented or delayed through guidance and intervention to reduce risk. Thus, it is important to know the risk factors for poor nutritional status in older persons and to intervene in a timely and appropriate fashion.

Inappropriate Food Intake

DEFINITION

Inappropriate food intake is inadequate or excessive consumption of food and fluid (nutrients).

REASON FOR CONCERN

To maintain optimal nutritional status, a person must have an appropriate food and fluid (nutrient) intake. People who are unable or unwilling to eat die unless fed via some other modality.[8,9] In the United States, the problem of overconsumption of food and fluid is of equal, if not greater, concern. Evidence that dietary excess contributes to several major chronic diseases that are leading causes of death in our society is strong and well documented.[1,4-6]

INTERVENTIONS

The frequency with which food is eaten, the quantity and quality of the food consumed, and other factors that contribute to excessive or inadequate food or fluid intake must be routinely and systematically assessed. Questions regarding programs that provide money for food, food itself, meals for the bedridden or infirm, or broader levels of economic, medical, or social support should be included. Direct observation of food intake, dietary recall or records of food intake, and careful questioning of both the older person and caregivers or family members are additional ways to gather information. Mistaken health beliefs, distorted body image, excessive prescribed or self-imposed dietary modifications should also be questioned. (See chapter 7 for additional information regarding assessment.)

Documentation of the data and its availability to appropriate members of the health care team is mandatory. Once specific problem areas are identified, appropriate nutritional, medical, social, and/or economic interventions can be implemented. These include, but are not limited to, dietary counseling, nutrition education, participation in food assistance or other community support programs, and implementation of dietary modifications or specialized feeding modalities. Longitudinal monitoring and appropriate modification of care plans developed are integral to this process.

Poverty

DEFINITION

Insufficient economic and other resources to meet basic needs define poverty. One hundred twenty-five percent of the federally designated "poverty level" in dollars is frequently used as the cutoff point for eligibility for a variety of service programs for the indigent.

REASON FOR CONCERN

Of the older adult population, approximately 10% of men and 30% of women report incomes of less than $5000 annually.[10] Low-income older adults often have limited access to food and limited food choices, particularly when utility and phone bills, medication, and similar expenses compete with their already scant funds.

National surveys of food consumption patterns show that low-income adults have consistently lower intakes of most nutrients.[5] The degree and significance of these findings depends on the specific nutrient assessed.

INTERVENTIONS

Questions regarding level and source(s) of income and adequacy of present income to meet basic needs must be asked whenever nutritional status is assessed. Questions regarding the specific amount of money or other resources available specifically for food may also yield significant information about the ability of older persons to obtain the food needed to maintain health. Reliance on any type of economic assistance program to meet basic needs (eg, food, housing, medical) should trigger an awareness that funds are limited and that risk of poor nutrition may be increased.

When a person's income is insufficient to meet basic needs, economic assistance can be sought on either an emergent or continuing basis. Food assistance and other similar services differ in availability and acceptability to the individual client. Awareness of the full range of options available increases the likelihood that identified needs will be met.

Social Isolation

DEFINITION

The Institute of Medicine defines social isolation as "the absence of social interactions, contacts, and relationships with family and friends, with neighbors on an individual level and with 'society at large' on a broader level."[1] Social isolation is usually measured by evaluating the type and strength of peoples' social support network and how they use it.

REASON FOR CONCERN

It is well documented that social interaction has a positive impact on health, quality of life, and food intake.[11-13] But as age increases, losses of family and friends are inevitable. Aging people often experience declines in independence, self-esteem, and income. Feelings of apathy, denial, depression, grief, loneliness, and/or suicidal rumination may be overwhelming. All of these have the potential to impact food intake and nutritional status negatively.

INTERVENTIONS

Attempts must be made to identify socially isolated people and to provide or to increase their opportunity for social interactions. It is particularly important for the dietetics professional to assess individual utilization of senior citizen centers, congregate feeding sites, meals-on-wheels programs, and similar community resources that supply food, promote social contact, and provide opportunities to use and maintain their interpersonal skills. Participation in such programs should be encouraged, when appropriate.

Physical Inactivity or Impaired Functional Status

DEFINITION

Physical inactivity or impaired functional status is defined as an inadequate level of aerobic fitness or an inability to perform those activities necessary for routine self-care.

REASON FOR CONCERN

It is estimated that at least one third of United States adults have extremely sedentary life-styles or inadequate levels of aerobic fitness.[2,14] Studies in men show that mortality due to all causes seems to increase as levels of physical activity decline.[15-18] On the other hand exercise appears to be especially effective for improving health in adults who have problems with coronary artery disease, hypertension, non-insulin-dependent diabetes mellitus, osteoporosis, and diminished psychological well-being.[14-17] Exercise for the elderly can increase opportunities for social contact and promote gains in cerebral function. In addition to the potential for improving health, exercise may also improve nutrient intake, improve sleep patterns, help to correct constipation, and delay or reverse the losses in lean body mass and bone mass associated with osteoporosis.[14-17]

Maintaining or improving the capacity to function and the potential to delay institutionalization may be the best reasons to encourage regular physical activity in older people. The prevalence of functional limitations in older adults living in the community increases with advancing age and is well described in other references.[1,2,7,19] Difficulty in performing the activities of daily living (ADL) or the instrumental activities of daily living (IADL) are often cited as factors in the decision to institutionalize.

INTERVENTIONS

A general indication of functional status is often useful in determining increased nutritional risk. Tools most often used to accomplish this task are the ADL and IADL assessment protocols.[20-23] It goes without saying that assessment of eating behavior and factors that contribute to eating dependency are also important. Difficulties related to eating, food preparation, or food procurement must be identified and documented early, and appropriate community or social service interventions, or therapeutic modalities, implemented.

Selected Acute and Chronic Diseases or Conditions

Diseases or conditions of particular concern that will be discussed here include alcohol abuse, constipation, dehydration, depression, oral health, protein-calorie malnutrition, and sensory impairment. The presence of any acute or chronic disease or condition, depending on the prior health and nutritional status of the person afflicted and the nature and the extent of the disease or conditions' effects, has the potential to negatively impact nutritional status. It is also well documented that hospitalization, trauma, surgery, and infection often have a negative impact upon nutritional health.[7-9] Complaints, clinical manifestations or symptoms of diet-related diseases, or decline in the ability to eat, prepare, or purchase food are all warning signs of increased nutritional risk.

Alcohol Abuse

DEFINITION

According to the Diagnostic and Statistical Manual of Mental Disorders,[24] there are three main patterns of alcohol abuse or dependence: regular daily intake of large amounts of alcohol; regular heavy drinking limited to weekends; and long periods of sobriety interspersed with binges of daily drinking lasting weeks or months. Although alcohol dependence is frequently associated with depression, depression appears to be the result of, rather than the cause of the drinking.

REASON FOR CONCERN

It is estimated that approximately 55% of US adults drink alcoholic beverages.[10] Approximately 11% to 13% of adults (21% of men) are considered heavy drinkers, consuming more than 60 drinks per month.[23,24] For those aged 65 years and older, current estimates of the prevalence of alcohol abuse range from 1% to 8% in the free-living population to 19% to 27% in hospital or nursing facility populations.[24-26] Estimates of direct health care costs related to alcohol abuse range from $10 billion to $15 billion annually.

The adverse effects of excessive alcohol on nutritional status are well documented. All organ systems may be affected.[17,27,28] Signs and symptoms include anemia, cardiac arrhythmias, cognitive impairment, confusion, edema, gastrointestinal bleeding, heart failure, hypertension, lipid disturbances, liver failure, malnutrition, osteoporosis, renal failure, trauma, and weight loss.

INTERVENTIONS

It is important to evaluate how often alcohol is consumed and whether this level of consumption represents a health hazard. Older people may show a different pattern of alcohol abuse than younger people. Differences in body composition and changes in metabolism that occur as part of the aging process may alter one's sensitivity to alcohol and intensify its deleterious effects.[24-29] The evaluation process uses easily administered, standardized questionnaires.[7,30,31]

Once a problem has been identified, dietetics professionals should work with other members of the health care team who are involved in the treatment process, to make them aware of the nutritional implications, and to correct nutritional deficits.

Constipation

DEFINITION

Constipation is the infrequent or difficult evacuation of feces.[32] People often subjectively define constipation as the passage of fewer than "normal" bowel movements and/or increased difficulty in defecation.[2] Because the range of normal for this bodily function varies, more precise definitions are lacking.

REASON FOR CONCERN

Constipation is not an inevitable part of the aging process, but physiologic alterations that sometimes accompany aging, such as decreased intestinal motility, increased transit time, and a decreased urge to defecate, may contribute to its prevalence. In older population groups, laxatives are one of the three most commonly purchased categories of nonprescription medications[33-35]; during the 1980s, approximately $38 billion was spent annually on laxatives.[2] So there is indirect evidence, at least, that the perception of real or imagined constipation in our population, particularly our ambulatory elderly population, is high.

Residents in nursing facilities experience frequent and often significant problems with constipation.[36] Common contributors to this problem are inadequate fiber or fluid intakes and immobility.[2,15] Diseases such as cancer, diabetes, and other neurologic or endocrine disorders contribute secondarily to this problem as do medications commonly prescribed or purchased over the counter.

Fecal impaction, overflow incontinence, obstruction, and terminal reservoir syndrome are potential outcomes of chronic, extreme constipation. Persons at high risk include those who are immobile, confused, or heavily medicated, particularly with drugs that have significant anticholinergic properties. Persons with systemic diseases such as uremia, hypothyroidism, or hypercalcemia may also experience significant problems with constipation. Changes in bowel habits often occur with diverticular disease and colon cancer.

INTERVENTIONS

Dietary modifications can be effective in the prevention or treatment of primary constipation. Increased dietary fiber and fluid intakes are recommended, as is regular physical activity. Medication protocols should be reviewed and less constipating alternatives recommended when appropriate. Systemic disease should, of course, be treated.

The dose of dietary fiber needed to improve bowel function is highly variable but is usually in the range of 6 to 10 g per day. Coarse wheat bran provides greatest fecal bulking capacity, and bulking agents such as psyllium, methylcellulose, carboxymethylcellulose, and polycarbophil produce laxative effects due to their water-holding properties and the mechanical distention of the gastrointestinal (GI) tract. These bulking agents are sometimes more acceptable than coarse wheat bran.[2]

The gradual introduction of high-fiber diets and fiber supplements over several weeks and in slowly increasing amounts helps to minimize flatulence, distention, and the abdominal discomfort that sometimes accompanies the introduction of high-fiber regimens. A variety of food sources of dietary fiber is preferred, but supplements can be used to augment them if the food sources fail to produce the desired effect when given an adequate trial.

People who have neuromuscular damage, adhesions due to prior surgeries, chronic disability, or chronic laxative abuse do not always respond to fiber therapy. However, these circumstances do not automatically preclude a trial of fiber therapy, bowel training, and other rehabilitative efforts.

Dehydration

DEFINITION

The condition that results from excessive loss of body water is dehydration.[32] However, "dehydration" is often more than a change in water balance since shifts in electrolyte balance occur as well.

REASON FOR CONCERN

Lean body mass and body water content decrease with age. Total body water decreases with age from approximately 60% to 45% of body weight.[26] There is a proportionate increase in body fat and less water reserves. Lower body reserves of water means a smaller volume of water for distribution of water-soluble substances such as alcohol and some drugs.[2] Dehydration may result from standard quantities or doses that are generally "safe" or recommended for adults. Diuretics and laxatives are of particular concern in this age group because their rate of use is so high.[33-35]

Declines in thirst perception, renal concentrating capacity, renal sodium-conserving capacity, and increases in antidiuretic hormone (ADH) secretion also contribute to increased risk of dehydration, especially when fluid intake is limited.[2,26] The presence of fever, diarrhea, vomiting, uncontrolled diabetes mellitus, and some forms of renal disease increase risk as well. Strenuous exercise or very hot weather may also precipitate problems.

Symptoms of dehydration in older persons include dryness of the lips or oral mucosa, turbidity of the tongue, sunken eyeballs, temperature elevation, hypotension, tachycardia, decreased urine output, constipation, nausea and vomiting, altered mental status, or confusion.[2,37] Often, these signs go unrecognized or are attributed to other causes.

INTERVENTIONS

Measures that may help prevent dehydration include informing older people of the signs of dehydration and encouraging appropriate fluid intakes, encouraging foods with low solute loads, and making fluids visible and readily available to older persons at home or in the nursing facility.

Fluid requirements are estimated at 1 mL/kcal ingested or 30 mL/kg body weight. When the volume deficit is modest (1L to 2L), it may be corrected by oral fluid intake, provided GI function and mental status are not impaired.[26] If oral rehydration is not possible or the volume deficit is large, intravenous therapy is indicated. (See chapter 6 for additional discussion.)

Depression

DEFINITION

The essential feature of major depressive disorder is either depressed mood or loss of interest in all, or almost all activities, for a period of at least 2 weeks.[24] If the altered mood represents a change from the previous level of functioning and if it persists, that may signal a major depressive disorder. Associated symptoms include appetite disturbance, change in weight, sleep disturbance, psychomotor agitation or retardation, decreased energy, feelings of worthlessness or excessive or inappropriate guilt, difficulty thinking or concentrating, and recurrent thoughts of death, or suicidal ideation or attempts. Associated features of depression include tearfulness, anxiety, irritability, brooding or obsessive rumination, excessive concern with physical health, panic attacks, and phobias.[24]

REASON FOR CONCERN

Although the prevalence of clinical depression in the general population is estimated at only 3% to 5%, 30% to 50% of adults report development of depression at some point during their lifetime. The costs incurred by persons with depression are greater than $16 billion annually.[7,17] In nursing facility populations, major depressive disorders occurred in 12.6% of patients, while 18.1% of patients experienced depressive symptoms.[38] Major depressive disorder is a significant risk factor for mortality and a 59% increased likelihood of death within 1 year of diagnosis.

Depression or the depressive disorders significantly impact quality of life. Level of function, productivity, and perceived physical and mental health are also impaired. Nutritional status is in jeopardy since so many of the signs and symptoms of depression relate to changes in appetite and weight, and lack of interest in food. In fact, depression has been shown to be a leading cause of unexplained weight loss in the elderly.[38,39]

The psychotropic drugs commonly used to treat depression such as antidepressants, antipsychotics, antianxiety agents, and anticholinergic agents can cause significant side effects and can negatively impact the ability to eat and, in turn, nutritional status. Oversedation, increased or decreased appetite, dry mouth, nausea, anorexia, and constipation—all common side effects of these drugs[40] may contribute to increased nutritional risk.

INTERVENTIONS

Numerous screening tools are available to determine emotional status including the Geriatric Depression Scale, Beck Depression Index, and others.[3,23,26] Although dietetic practitioners do not typically administer these instruments, the registered dietitian nevertheless should be cognizant of their content, use, and implications. Changes in mood, attitude, or level of performance should alert all dietetics professionals to the potential for depression. Discussion of this possibility with other members of the health care team is appropriate, as is periodic inquiry into the resident's emotional status.

The regular review of medications prescribed to treat depression is indicated in light of their potential negative impact on the older person's ability to eat. Drug-free trials or reductions in dosages should be recommended, particularly if these agents appear to be a source of significant nutritional impairment.

Oral Health Problems

DEFINITION

Tooth loss, dental caries, lack of or poorly fitting dentures, periodontal disease, pathologies of the oral tissues, dry mouth, and orofacial pain are oral health problems.[2,7]

REASON FOR CONCERN

Problems with the oral cavity often impair one's ability to eat. Local as well as systemic morbidity may result; decreases in life satisfaction abound.[41] Although recent data from national surveys suggest that older people retain their teeth for a longer period,[41,42] the prevalence of oral cancer, cervical (root) caries, and edentulism increases with advancing age. Oral cancer accounts for approximately 4% of all cancer and 2.4% of cancer deaths annually.[17,42] The majority of these deaths occur in persons over age 65.

A major cause of unexplained weight loss in older persons is oral health problems. As the number of dental problems increases, so does the rate of weight loss. Taste, chewing, and swallowing may also be impaired in persons with oral health problems. Diminished taste or alterations in taste perception are often experienced by persons with complete dentures.[43]

INTERVENTIONS

Periodic examination of the oral tissues and documentation of findings is mandatory. Appropriate intervention has the potential to significantly improve food intake, nutritional status, and to enhance quality of life.

Protein-Energy Malnutrition

DEFINITION

Protein-energy malnutrition (PEM) is characterized by wasting and excessive loss of lean body mass resulting from too little energy or protein being supplied to body tissues.[2,44] PEM is an indicator of, rather than a risk factor for, poor nutritional status. However, malnourished people are certainly at increased risk of morbidity and mortality.[8,9,44]

REASON FOR CONCERN

In the ambulatory, noninstitutionalized older population, the prevalence of PEM is low, probably less than 1%.[2] However, risk of PEM is probably high, particularly in those persons with inadequate access to food, or with chronic diseases or conditions that predispose them to marginal nutrient intakes. Incidence of malnutrition in hospitalized and nursing facility populations is high and varies according to the criteria used to assess nutritional status.[2,44,45]

The health consequences of PEM are serious and well documented.[2,8,9,37,44] These include: loss of lean body mass, decreased muscle strength, increased susceptibility to infection, decline in functional status, increased confusion and other behavioral abnormalities, a propensity for the development of pressure ulcers, increased complication rates postsurgery and during the treatment of coexisting disease, and, if PEM is severe, premature death. Altered drug metabolism and increased drug toxicity may also result from PEM.[2,26,44]

INTERVENTIONS

Screening for PEM can help to identify high-risk persons and allow caregivers to institute preventive measures before a deficiency becomes clinically apparent.[22,23,46] A careful history or chart review may be sufficient to detect PEM. If the results are inconclusive and the level of suspicion is high, further physical examination or laboratory evaluation is justified[44] (see chapter 6).

Sensory Impairment

DEFINITION

Sensory impairment is the abnormal, diminished, delayed or lack of perception, or response to stimuli.

REASON FOR CONCERN

Functional changes in sensory organs occur with advancing age and are associated with increased risk of poor nutritional status.[12] Declines in hearing and vision are among the ten most common conditions reported by persons aged 65 years and older.[47] Marked declines in taste and smell may also be experienced. The perception of sweet and salty tastes seems to be affected first, while the perception of sour and bitter tastes remains.

Peripheral neuropathies and other tactile impairments may also negatively impact nutritional status. Food preparation becomes more difficult, increasing the likelihood of burns or other injuries.[7]

The appearance and crispness or crunchiness of a food can often make up for some taste or smell deficits. If all of the senses are diminished, however, food intake decreases and, as a consequence, social contact declines—another reason for concern.

INTERVENTIONS

The use of flavor and odor enhancers in food products for the elderly is a novel approach to this problem. Such strategies are being implemented on a limited basis around the country.[48,49] Bright, contrasting colors in foods, plates, and eating utensils, and well-lit dining areas may also stimulate increased food intake. Hearing-impaired adults may be reluctant to eat in noisy, crowded dining rooms, or at large tables because they cannot enjoy mealtime conversations and feel isolated. Recognition of these factors and modification of the older person's eating environment may facilitate improved food intake (see chapter 8).

Chronic or Inappropriate Use of Medications

DEFINITION

The long-term use of prescribed or over-the-counter (OTC) medications describes chronic medication use. Inappropriate medication use refers to medications prescribed or consumed in such a manner that dose, type, or other characteristics are incompatible with the physiology (including the nutritional status) or psychology of the aging person.[2]

REASON FOR CONCERN

The potential is high for inappropriate use of medications or for drug-nutrient or drug-drug interactions with negative impact upon nutritional status in older population groups. In non-nursing home settings, it has been shown that 27% of older persons take at least one medication and 23% take at least five. The rest take between two and five medications daily. In elderly nursing facility populations, 45% take at least five or more drugs daily and everyone takes at least one.[50] In one study, combined prescribed and OTC drug use by ambulatory elderly averaged 7.9 drugs per person per day.[51]

Cardiovascular agents represent between 54% to 75% of all drugs prescribed for the elderly. This drug category includes diuretics, antihypertensives, antiarrhythmics, cardiac glycosides, potassium supplements, anticoagulants, and vasodilators.[34,35] The next three most frequently prescribed drug categories are central nervous system agents (antidepressant, antipsychotic, antiseizure medications), analgesics (nonsteroidal anti-inflammatory agents, narcotics), and endocrine and metabolic agents (oral hypoglycemics).[35] Nonprescription drugs most frequently used by older persons are analgesics (aspirin, acetaminophen), nutritional supplements (vitamins, minerals), and GI agents (laxatives, antacids).[35]

INTERVENTIONS

The potential for both prescribed and OTC drugs to impact nutritional status negatively is well documented.[2,7,40,50] Dietetics professionals must be constantly alert to the possibility of drug-nutrient interactions. They also must be well versed in the effects these drugs have on nutritional status and be ready to intervene early in the course of treatment.

Drugs accounting for the largest percentages of potential problems in the elderly are the cardiac glycosides, furosemide, oral hypoglycemics, antacids, beta blockers, thiazide diuretics, phenytoin sodium, cimetadine, and aspirin.[40,51] The nutritional impact of these drugs is described in other references.[2,7,40,50] Drug-food and drug-alcohol incompatibilities also are recognizable and preventable in most instances.[40]

Summary

It is important to view each older person as a unique individual with a unique set of nutrition needs and concerns.[7] Although functional impairment and progressive disability tend to increase with age, generalizations regarding the care of specific elderly people are, for the most part, inappropriate. Familiarity with the resident's unique circumstances and requirements, as well as routine surveillance and continuity of care, offer the most promise for prompt identification of increased risk and timely and appropriate nutrition intervention. Through such practices, optimal, achievable nutritional health will be maintained.

References

1. Institute of Medicine. *The Second Fifty Years: Promoting Health and Preventing Disability*. Washington, DC: National Academy Press; 1990.
2. Dwyer JT. *Screening Older Americans' Nutritional Health—Current Practices and Future Possibilities*. Washington, DC: Nutrition Screening Initiative; 1991.
3. White JV, Ham RJ, Lipschitz DA, Dwyer JT, Wellman NS. Consensus of the Nutrition Screening Initiative: risk factors and indicators of poor nutritional status in older Americans. *J Am Diet Assoc*. 1991;91:783-787.
4. *The Surgeon General's Report on Nutrition and Health*. Washington, DC: US Dept of Health and Human Services, Public Health Services, US Government Printing Office; 1988. DHHS publication (PHS)88-S0210.
5. National Research Council. *Diet and Health: Implications for Reducing Chronic Disease Risk*. Washington, DC: National Academy of Sciences; 1989.
6. *Healthy People 2000: National Health Promotion and Disease Prevention Objectives*. Washington, DC: US Dept of Health and Human Services; 1990.
7. White JV. Risk factors for poor nutritional status in older Americans. *Am Fam Physician*. 1991;44:2087-2097.

8.   Bistrian BR, Blackburn GL, Vitale J, Cochran D, Naylor J. Prevalence of malnutriton in general medical patients. *JAMA.* 1976;235:1576.

9.   Cahill GF. Starvation in man. *N Engl J Med.* 1970;282:668-675

10. *Statistical Abstract of the United States: 1991.* 111th ed. Washington, DC: US Bureau of the Census; 1991.

11. Ryan KC, Bower ME. Relationship of socioeconomic status and living arrangements to nutritional intake of the older person. *J Am Diet Assoc.* 1989;89:1805-1807.

12. Hickler RB, Wayne KS. Nutrition and the elderly. *Am Fam Physician* 1984;29:137-145.

13. Walker D, Beauchene RE. The relationship of loneliness, social isolation and physical health to dietary adequacy of independent living elderly. *J Am Diet Assoc.* 1991;91:300-304.

14. Casperson CJ, Christenson GM, Pollard RA. Status of the 1990 physical fitness and exercise objectives: evidence from NH15 1985. *Public Health Rep.* 1986;101:587-592.

15. Shephard RJ. The scientific basis for exercise prescribing for the very old. *J Am Geriatr Soc.* 1990;38:62-70.

16. Paffenbarger RS, Hyde RT, Wing AL, Hsiek CC. Physical activity, all-cause mortality and longevity of college alumni. *N Engl J Med.* 1986;314:605-613

17. US Preventive Services Task Force. *Guide to Clinical Preventive Services: an assessment of the effectiveness of 169 interventions.* Baltimore, Md: Williams and Wilkins; 1989.

18. Leon AS, Connett J, Jacobs DR, Rauramaa R. Leisure-time physical activity levels and risk of coronary heart disease and death. The Multiple Risk Factor Intervention Trial. *JAMA.* 1987; 258:2388-2395.

19. Dawson D, Hendershot G, Fulton J. Aging in the eighties: functional limitations of individuals age 65 years and over. In: *Advance Data from Vital and Health Statistics of the National Center for Health Statistics, 133.* Rockville, Md; US Dept of Health and Human Services, Public Health Service; 1987.

20. Katz S, Downs TD, Cash HR. Progress in the development of the index of ADL. *Gerontol.* 1970;10:20-30.

21. Lawton MP, Brody EM. Assessment of older people: self-monitoring and instrumental activities of daily living. *Gerontol.* 1969;9:179-186.

22. White JV, Dwyer JT, Posner BM, Ham RJ, Lipschitz DA, Wellman NS. Nutrition Screening Initiative: development and implementation of the public awareness checklist and screening tools. *J Am Diet Assoc.* 1992; 92:163-167.

23. *Nutrition Screening Manual for Professionals Caring for Older Americans.* Washington, DC: Nutrition Screening Initiative: 1991.

24. American Psychiatric Association. *Diagnostic and Statistical Manual of Mental Disorders, Third Edition—Revised.* Washington, DC: American Psychiatric Association; 1987.

25. Kamerow DB, Pincus HA, Macdonald DT. Alcohol abuse, other drug abuse and mental disorders in medical practice: prevalence, costs, recognition and treatment. *JAMA.* 1986;255:2054-2057.

26. *The Merck Manual of Geriatrics.* Rahway, NJ: Merck and Co; 1990.

27. Willenbring ML. Organic and mental disorders associated with binge drinking and alcohol dependence. *Clin Geriatr Med.* 1988;4:869-888.

28. Goodwin JS. Social, psychological and physical factors affecting the nutritional status of elderly subjects: separating cause and effect. *Am J Clin Nutr.* 1989;50:1201-1209.

29. Adams WL, Gary PH, Rhyne R, Hunt WC, Goodwin JS. Alcohol intake in the healthy elderly: changes with age in a cross-sectional and longitudinal study. *J Am Geriatr Soc.* 1990;38:211-216.

30. Willenbring MC, Spring WD. Evaluating alcohol use in elders. *Q J Am Soc Aging.* 1988;12:27-31.
31. US Preventive Services Task Force Report. Screening for alcohol and other drug abuse. Am Fam Physician. 1989;40:137-146.
32. *Dorland's Illustrated Medical Dictionary.* 27th ed. Philadelphia, Pa: WB Saunders Co; 1988.
33. May FE, Stewart RB, Hale WE, Marks RG. Prescribed and non prescribed drug use in an ambulatory elderly population. *South Med J.* 1982;75:522-528.
34. Hale WE, May FE, Marks RG, Stewart RB. Drug use in an ambulatory elderly population: a five year update. *Drug Intell Clin Pharm.* 1987;21:530-535.
35. Helling DK, Lemke JH, Selma TP, Wallace RB, Lipson DP, Cornoni-Huntley J. Medication use characteristics in the elderly: the Iowa 65 + rural health study. *J Am Geriatr Soc.* 1987;35:4-12.
36. Alessi CA, Henderson CT. Constipation and fecal impaction in the long term care patient. *Clin Geriatr Med.* 1988;4:571-588.
37. Chernoff R, Lipschitz DA. Nutrition and aging. In: Shils ME, Young VR, eds. *Modern Nutrition in Health and Disease.* 7th ed. Philadelphia, Pa: Lea & Febiger; 1988.
38. Rovner BW, German PS, Brant LJ, Clark R, Burton L, Folstein MF. Depression and mortality in nursing homes. *JAMA.* 1991;265:993-996.
39. Thompson MP, Morris LK. Unexplained weight loss in the ambulatory elderly. *J Am Geriatr Soc.* 1991;39:497-500.
40. Kurfees JF, Dotson RL. Drug interactions in the elderly. *J Fam Pract.* 1987;25:477-488.
41. Dolan TA, Monopoli, MP, Kaurich MJ, Rubenstein LZ. Geriatric grand rounds: oral disease in older adults. *J Am Geriatr Soc.* 1990;38:1239-1250.
42. *Oral Health of United States Adults. The National Survey of Oral Health in US Employed Adults and Seniors: 1985-86, National Findings.* Washington, DC: US Dept of Health and Human Services; 1987. NIH publication 87-2868.
43. Papas AS, Palmer CA, Rounds MC, et al. Longitudinal relationships between nutrition and oral health. *Ann NY Acad Sci.* 1989;561:124-142.
44. Ham RJ. Indicators of poor nutritional status in older Americans. *Am Fam Physician.* 1992;45:219-228.
45. Pinchcofsky-Devin GD, Kaminski MV. Incidence of protein calorie malnutrition in the nursing home population. *J Am Coll Nutr.* 1987;6:109-112.
46. Lipschitz DA, Ham RJ, White JV. An approach to nutrition screening for older Americans. *Am Fam Physician.* 1992;45: In press.
47. Collins, JG. Prevalence of selected chronic conditions, United States, 1983-85. In: *Advance Data from Vital and Health Statistics of the National Center for Health Statistics, 155.* Rockville, Md: US Dept of Health and Human Services, Public Health Service; 1988.
48. Wysocki CJ, Gilbert AN. National geographic smell survey: effects of age are heterogenous. *Ann NY Acad Sci.* 1989;561:12-28.
49. Bartoshuk LM. Taste: robust across the age span? *Ann NY Acad Sci.* 1989;561:87-93.
50. Lamay PP, Michocki RJ. Medication management. *Clin Geriatr Med.* 1988;4:623-638.
51. Darnell JC, Murra MD, Martz BL, Weinberger M. Medication use in an ambulatory elderly population: an in-home survey. *J. Am Geriatr Soc.* 1986;34:1-4.

4. QUALITY OF LIFE

Liberalized Approach to Nutrient Modification

Residents' Rights and Responsibilities Related to Nutrition Care

Registered Dietitian's Responsibilities Related to Resident Care

Position of The American Dietetic Association: Issues in Feeding the Terminally Ill Adult

4. Quality of Life

Grow old along with me!
The best is yet to be,
The last of life, for which the first was made.
                    Robert Browning

The obligation of registered dietitians and professional caregivers is to ensure and enhance the quality of life for each resident in the nursing facility by providing appropriate nutrition care and by recognizing and honoring the individuality of each person.

Quality of life issues are emphasized throughout the Omnibus Budget Reconciliation Act (OBRA) of 1987 by giving the resident the power of choice. The quality of life regulation reads:

> A facility must care for its residents in a manner and in an environment that promotes maintenance or enhancement of each resident's quality of life.

The OBRA regulations focus on the delivery of care and the results of that care. The registered dietitian has the opportunity to be proactive in assessing the needs of residents, in delivering high quality nutritional care, and in eliminating or reducing malnutrition . . . . This is an excellent time to let administrators know why a registered dietitian's services are important to the health and nutritional status of residents in long term care facilities." [1]

Among numerous factors to consider in nutrition care for the elderly are: an understanding of the ethnic, social, and economic eating patterns that influence the resident's way of life; medical coverage available; and limited budget. Other contributing factors include emotional, physical, and biological changes in the resident's life-style, including the loss of a spouse, separation from family and friends, leaving home and job, decreased mobility, financial limitation, and loss of independence. Previous chapters have discussed in detail the relationship of nutrition and disease in the older person and risk factors associated with poor nutritional status. There are also unavoidable effects of aging that can combine to rob a resident of the simple pleasure of eating. These conditions can also increase the risk of compromising nutritional status. Sensory changes in taste, smell, hearing, sight, and touch diminish the resident's enjoyment of meals. Frequently, favorite foods of the past no longer have the same appeal. Lack of strength often causes a weakened ability to grasp and hold utensils and dishes. Impaired vision reduces appetite stimulation and anticipation of a pleasurable meal. Depression can decrease the desire to eat and cause anorexia.[2-5] These impairments are necessarily considerations when planning nutrition services to meet nutrition needs and maintain or enhance a resident's quality of life.

It is an exciting time for registered dietitians to provide positive, creative approaches to managing the nutrition care of residents in nursing facilities. The challenge is to be aware of the things that are important to the elderly and to consider their happiness and peace of mind within the framework of rules and regulations. Serving attractive meals on schedule in a pleasant, relaxed atmosphere, and allowing adequate time to eat and to socialize with other residents enhances the general well-being of the elderly. This is the kind of environment that maximizes the quality of life and preserves the dignity of the individual.[2]

Liberalized Approach to Nutrient Modification

A diet order that imposes many restrictions can contribute significantly to reduced food intake and a marked decline in a resident's nutritional status. With the denial of favorite foods or the enforcement of a strange diet, the resident's quality of life is diminished even further. Over the past decade many health professionals have encouraged dietitians to simplify and liberalize modified diets.[6]

According to research into the process of aging and disease, a well-balanced diet is the key factor in maintaining good health. Unless the resident eats the food served, no benefit is derived. Restrictive diets add to the resident's already existing problems. Valid nutrition practices in the use of sound nutrition information must be included in dietary management for the nursing facility resident to combat the nutritional misconceptions of the resident, the resident's family, and the staff.

Through years of experience, many registered dietitians have found a regular diet to be the most appropriate one for the majority of elderly residents. Of course, certain medical conditions require diet modifications, but these usually can be met with simple adjustments and minimal restrictions.

In recommending a therapeutic diet, the physician should carefully weigh the potential benefits against the possible detriments to optimal food intake and the disruption in the resident's quality of life. The probable consequences of restricting certain foods must be considered. The resulting stress (anger, anxiety, depression) may be more damaging than the food itself. Two questions should be answered before imposing a restrictive modified diet: "Will the diet contribute to overall health and quality of life, or will it lead to loss of appetite and malnutrition instead? Are the resident's rights being acknowledged, or is he or she being deprived of familiar, well-liked foods for reasons that are vaguely defined?" [4]

Registered dietitians in different areas of the country share similar results when reporting on the implementation of liberalized diets in nursing facilities. They report no significant changes in blood pressure, weight, blood glucose, or edema following the removal of most restrictions. Most residents' needs are met by planning a well-balanced, regular diet to meet individual nutrition needs and personal food preferences. Removing salt packets or table salt from a resident requiring sodium restriction is usually adequate. For control of non-insulin-dependent diabetes, a regular diet with limited concentrated sweets and no sugar packet meets the needs of most diabetic residents. Many positive results are demonstrated with a liberalized approach to nutrient modification. A resident generally is more satisfied with a variety of food choices, compliance improves, and there is contentment in having favorite foods. A regular diet with slight modifications generally is recommended and encouraged to ensure adequate calorie intake and maximize the pleasure of eating. Be careful not to restrict particular foods in the name of good nutrition care. Food is not nutritious unless consumed.[2,4]

John E. Morley, MB, BCh, of St Louis University's, Division of Geriatric Medicine, states, "Don't try to change life-style eating habits in the nursing home. Give them what allowed them to get to their 70s and 80s and (what will allow them) to enjoy their twilight years." [5]

Residents' Rights and Responsibilities Related to Nutrition Care

All residents in nursing facilities have rights guaranteed to them under federal and state law. Requirements concerning resident rights are specified under Federal Regulations 483.10, 483.12, 483.13, and 483.15.

The following is a list of residents' rights and responsibilities relating to nutrition care.

A resident has the right:[7]

- To be treated with dignity and self-respect.
- To receive reasonable accommodation of individual needs and preferences, except when health or safety or the health and safety of other residents would be endangered.
- To choose activities, schedules, and health care consistent with individual interests, assessments, and plan of care.
- To be served nourishing, palatable, well-balanced meals that meet daily nutrition and special needs.
- To be served food according to ethnic, cultural, or religious customs.
- To make choices about where, when, and what to eat.
- To be provided adequate fluids to maintain proper hydration and care.
- To participate in the planning of menus and special meals as desired.
- To have meals served in a cheerful, relaxed, quiet, pleasant surrounding that is well-lighted, ventilated, adequately furnished, and has sufficient space for safety and comfort.
- To be encouraged and allowed to remain independent in feeding oneself.

- To be provided with adaptive eating devices to assist in maintaining independence in eating.
- To receive assistance, encouragement, and prompting during a meal as appropriate to ensure adequate nutritional intake.
- To receive prompt assistance with feeding when the meal is served if unable to feed oneself.
- To a dignified dining setting regardless of ability to feed oneself. A resident with dysphagia should have the same dining atmosphere as other residents.
- To be allowed time to complete meals without feeling rushed.
- To be served food that has been prepared under sanitary conditions and served at the proper temperature.
- To be provided texture of food at highest level tolerated. This may mean varying the texture at different meals depending on resident's alertness, fatigue, particular food item, or personal preference.
- To be served attractive, well-seasoned food in portions acceptable.
- To be offered substitutes of similar nutritive value when food served is refused.
- To have availability of seconds on food if desired and allowed.
- To be served within a reasonable time of scheduled meal services.
- To participate in choosing dining companions to enhance socialization during meals.
- To be seated at a table of appropriate height for proper positioning.
- To be taken to the dining room appropriately groomed (hair combed, face and hands washed) and clothed.
- To receive additional nutrition support appropriate for maintaining acceptable parameters of nutritional status, such as body weight and protein levels, unless the resident's clinical condition demonstrates it is not possible.
- To receive a therapeutic diet when there is a medical problem dictating adjustment from the regular diet.
- To receive necessary nutrition support to promote healing, and prevent infection of pressure ulcers, and to prevent new sores from developing.
- To receive the appropriate treatment and services to prevent aspiration pneumonia, diarrhea, vomiting, dehydration, metabolic abnormalities, and nasopharyngeal ulcers when nasogastric or gastrostomy tube feeding is required to provide adequate nutrition.
- To have access to caregivers that provide nutrition services.
- To voice complaints and concerns regarding the food, meal service, or any other aspect of nutrition care without fear of reprisal.
- To receive consultation concerning nutrition information and instruction relating to needs and interests.
- To expect the correct interpretation of orders and delivery of nutrition services to meet needs and preferences.
- To refuse any part or all nutrition treatment.

A resident has the responsibility:
- To follow the nutrition care plan recommended by the registered dietitian.
- To seek more nutrition information and/or clarification of information given if questions remain, and request follow-up.
- For the adverse consequences if the nutrition care plan and/or diet as outlined is refused.

Registered Dietitian Responsibilities Related to Resident Care

The registered dietitian should have plans that cover a complete range of nutrition services for residents. The following are examples of services the registered dietitian performs to ensure a high level of continuous quality improvement (CQI):
- Provides direction in implementation of the nutrition components of the care plan by communicating with the professional staff and by data collection.
- Promotes communications (written and verbal) and public relations inter- and intradepartmentally.
- Implements procedures for obtaining data collection needed to complete the nutrition assessment and care plan.
- Assists in the development of screening tools to assist the dietetic technician or dietary manager and professional staff in identifying residents requiring nutrition intervention.
- Develops protocols for residents at nutritional risk.
- Reviews, writes, or assists in writing menus that meet the current Recommended Dietary Allowances and reflect resident preferences. At a minimum, menus must be reviewed and revised biannually.
- Develops therapeutic diets and diets to meet the specialized needs of residents.
- Provides recommendations to the physician for appropriate diet orders that include enteral or parenteral feedings.
- Assesses the resident's need for special eating devices with consultation from the other professional staff.
- Provides direction for the nutrition component of discharge planning, including diet instruction and information about community programs.
- Provides continuing education programs for dietary staff.
- Conducts the nutrition education for nursing personnel at least annually.
- Selects and approves a current (5-year) diet manual appropriate to the needs of the facility.
- Develops an efficient system for transmitting and implementing diet orders and changes from nursing service to the dietary department.
- Monitors and evaluates food preparation and service for acceptability, taste, appearance, and portion size; makes recommendations as needed.

- Participates in budget preparation for the dietary department to ensure that staffing, food, and supplies are adequate for resident needs.
- Evaluates and makes recommendations for the adequacy and use of available equipment to provide the required food preparation and service.
- Provides guidance on the development of job specifications and descriptions, work schedules, and other management tools necessary for the efficient functioning of the dietary department.
- Develops and monitors sanitation and safety policies with procedures to ensure the safe storage, preparation, distribution, and service of food.
- Provides direction or develops guidelines for the dietetic component of the quality improvement program.

The registered dietitian should not be limited to providing these examples of service, but should also recommend a range of services to meet the nursing facility's nutrition needs.

It is important to remember that a consultant does not have actual authority. Administration is responsible for the overall operation of the facility: financial; personnel; adhering to rules, regulations, and laws; and overall quality improvement of nutrition care.

To be an effective consultant and to achieve high quality nutrition care for each resident, it is imperative to develop a close working relationship with the administrator, the dietetic technician or dietary manager and members of the health care team.

References

1. ADA Division of Government Affairs. OBRA '87 update. *Legislative Newsletter.* Sept 30, 1991.
2. Coe DH, Hiett ES, Peterson MD. The quality of life diet guide. Englewood, Colo: Quality of Life Associates; 1990.
3. Davies L, Knutson KC. Warning signals for malnutrition in the elderly. J Am Diet Assoc. 1991; 91:1413–1417.
4. Opheim C, Wesselman J. Optimal dietary prescribing in the nursing home. *Geriatrics.* 1990;45:66–71.
5. Morley JE. Institutionalized death by starvation. Presented at the 74th Annual Meeting of The American Dietetic Association. Dallas, Tex; Oct 1991.
6. Lan SJ, Justice CL. Use of modified diets in nursing homes. J Am Diet Assoc. 1991;91:46–51.
7. Weerts S. Food rights of the elderly. *Consultant Dietitian.* 1990; 15:4.

Position of The American Dietetic Association: Issues in Feeding the Terminally Ill Adult

"Issues in feeding the terminally ill adult" identifies some of the ethical, legal, medical, and nutrition issues to be considered when deciding to provide or forgo nutrition support. The primary consideration in any decision must be the wishes of the competent, informed patient or his/her surrogate decision maker. Although each situation must be resolved individually, the paper does provide some considerations and questions to assist in developing an appropriate nutrition care plan.

Health care literature contains wide differences of opinion regarding decisions of whether to require or forgo life-sustaining procedures, including nutrition support, for a dying patient. The task requires sensitivity and wisdom. Strides have already been made to promote the use of rational, systematic procedures to determine appropriate types and levels of nutrition care for terminally ill adults.[1-7]

Position Statement

It is the position of The American Dietetic Association that the dietitian take an active role in developing criteria for feeding the terminally ill adult within the practice setting and collaborate with the health care team in making recommendations on each case.

Dietitians, like all other health care practitioners, are responsible for their own conduct. Terminally ill adults, like other competent individuals, have a right to be a major force in choosing which level of treatment and care they receive.[7-9] The dietitian, as part of the health care team, has a responsibility to meet the psychological and physiological needs and wants of each patient on an individualized basis.

This paper addresses some of the issues involved in feeding the terminally ill adult from ethical, legal, medical, and nutrition perspectives, concluding with specific considerations for deciding appropriateness of providing or withholding nutrition support.

DEFINITION OF TERMS

For purposes of this paper, the following terms will be used to mean:
- Terminal illness—the end or final stage of a specific, progressive, normally irreversible lethal disease when physicians have "determined, through objective medical validation, that medical treatment of that disease is futile"[3] and the disease will cause the patient's death in the foreseeable future.
- Death—the "irreversible cessation of cardiac and respiratory functions or irreversible cessation of all functions of the entire brain, including the brain stem." A determination of death must be made in accordance with accepted medical standards by a physician.[3]

■ Patient competence—legally interpreted as sufficient mental ability to understand a procedure or therapy, be able to weigh its risks and benefits, make a decision based on rational reasons and personal values, and comprehend the consequences of consenting to or refusing treatment.[8,10,11]

■ Ethical—pertaining to the rational processes for determining the most morally desirable course of action in the face of conflicting value choices.[11]

■ Legal—based upon or authorized by law.

Discussion of Ethical, Legal, Medical, and Nutrition Considerations for Feeding the Terminally Ill Adult

ETHICAL CONSIDERATIONS

The dietitian, like other health care professionals, has an inherent ethical responsibility to respect the sanctity of life and the dignity and rights of all persons and to provide relief from suffering.[8,9,12-18] Is it ethically defensible to forgo or discontinue hydration and nutrition support from any patient? The Council on Ethical and Judicial Affairs of the American Medical Association (AMA) answered this question affirmatively for some terminally ill as well as some persistent vegetative state (PVS) patients.[6] Health care literature contains many differences of opinion regarding the answer to this quandary.[1,7,19-29] "Radically different ethical conclusions are reached and are based on radically different fundamental ethical theories and methods of ethical reasoning."[17]

The most powerful ethical principle to consider is the patient's right of self-determination. Each patient approaches that universal, common end called death with different religious, philosophical, and personal attitudes and values. For some, every moment of life—no matter how painful and limited in quality—is of inestimable value.[30,31] Suffering may be perceived as an important means of personal growth or a religious experience.[17,18] Some patients may hope beyond medical prediction that, if they hold on long enough, a medical miracle cure will be discovered for their disease.[31] The legal, medical, and population majority opinion is that "neurological brain death" is a definition of death. However, a minority of specific groups or individuals, based on religious beliefs, do not accept the neurological criterion as the definition of death.[32] It is the dietitian's responsibility to provide a combination of emotional support and technical nutrition advice on how to best achieve each patient's goals within legal parameters.

On the other hand, because of their circumstances and values, competent, informed patients may seek to forgo various medical procedures—which may include nutrition support. Such interventions may be perceived as inhumane means of prolonging the emotional and physical suffering at the conclusion of life.[3,6,24] The fear of physical or emotional abandonment is among the most frequently cited apprehensions of the dying.[30,33] Assuming the patient continues to reject all forms of nutrition support, the dietitian must remain emotionally supportive of the patient.[2,23,33] Patients should always have the option and the opportunity to change their minds. The rejection of food should not be construed by the dietitian as a sign of personal or professional failure.

At the same time, health care professionals must be aware of personal factors that could interfere with the execution of their professional responsibilities. It is important for dietitians to be aware of their personal values and attitudes, in addition to having a clear understanding of the principles of The Commission on Dietetic Registration, The American Dietetic Association's code of ethics,[12] guidelines from the Joint Commission on Accreditation of Hospitals and Hospice Standards,[34] institutional guidelines, and sources of public policy. Respect for a patient's right of self-determination may result in a conflict with the dietitian's ethical value system. Some dietitians may believe that all patients are required to receive nutrition support; therefore, a patient's informed decision to forgo nutrition intervention might violate an individual dietitian's personal perception of professional responsibility.[15,16,24] Depending on the specifics of the situation, the dietitian has a number of options in resolving this ethical dilemma.

One approach is collaborative decision-making[16]:

1. Define the problem. What is the specific ethical dilemma? Is there a difference of opinion on the medical facts or nutrition management? What ethics, either personal or professional, are being potentially compromised by the decision?

2. Gather relevant data. This includes objective and subjective data pertinent to the patient, ie, diagnostic evaluation. Validate the analysis of the problem with authoritative citations.

3. Discuss the problem with others. This should include the patient, guardian, physician, nurse, administrator, and other health care professionals. When pertinent, legal counsel may be consulted. Present the perceived problem in a clear, well-organized, logical, succinct, nonhostile manner.

4. Decide what to do. Be able to validate basis for recommended decision.

   - Reevaluate the perceived dilemma in light of discussions and the overall view and purpose of the institution as well as local law, and available durable power of attorney for health care decisions.

   - If conflict is unresolved because of the dietitian's perceived personal or professional values, withdraw from the case provided arrangements have been made for continuous care by another dietitian.[3,15,22] Do not abandon the patient!

   - If the problem is perceived as a critical ethical/moral dilemma, consider taking the problem to a higher administrative authority. This may involve referral to the institution's ethics committee. In some instances, notification of legal authorities may be warranted.[7-9,12,16]

In all cases, respect and consideration for the patient's informed preference for the level of nutrition care is paramount.

LEGAL CONSIDERATIONS

How legally significant are the patient's opinions on setting limits for treatment options? What is the legal duty of health care facilities and professionals in providing nutrition support for the terminally ill adult? Is providing nourishment an integral part of mandatory palliative care or an optional medical treatment? Is iatrogenic malnutrition or dehydration grounds for a professional negligence lawsuit? Does a mentally competent adult have the right to refuse nutrition support? If an adult is not competent to decide, under what circumstances, if any, can a surrogate demand that artificial nutrition be discontinued? Does the physician or health care facility ever have the right to forcibly feed a competent adult over that adult's objections?

Although there are no simple, hard, fast rules to apply, awareness of pertinent legal doctrines of professional negligence and informed consent as illustrated by case law and statutes can provide insight into dealing with these difficult questions. Landmark court cases are presented to clarify these critical legal concepts. Although ADA's position addresses "terminally ill patients," cases involving other feeding cases are presented for their legal reasoning.

In the past decade, there has been a continuous flow of landmark judicial decisions addressing the issue of when life-sustaining procedures, such as kidney dialysis,[35] resuscitation,[36] respiratory support,[37] and now nutrition support,[5,38-45] can be immediately withdrawn or forgone. The topic has stimulated much public debate. It is beyond the scope of this position to present more than an overview of some of the most important issues within the topic. Extensive reading and discussion of the subject are recommended. Legal counsel can provide information on patients' rights and professional obligations.

Professional negligence. Dietitians, like physicians, health care administrators, and insurance companies, are apprehensive about possible malpractice claims. In the 1970s, Butterworth and Blackburn[46] brought professional and public attention to "iatrogenic malnutrition—the skeleton in the hospital closet." It should be remembered, however, that the medical and nutrition goals are frequently different for the terminally ill than for the acutely and chronically ill population.[15] (See sections on "Medical considerations" and "Nutrition considerations" for guidelines for standards of quality care.)

Informed consent. The most significant legal issue to be considered involves the informed competent patient's legal right to voluntarily consent to or refuse medical treatment. In most jurisdictions, failure to obtain informed consent from a patient is viewed as a form of medical negligence or malpractice. Generally, the standard used to assess whether the patient has received sufficient medical information is what other physicians do under similar circumstances. Instead of informational needs being measured by the hypothetical "reasonable patient" standard, more attention is being given to informational needs of an "actual, specific patient."[8] Effective December 1, 1991, the Patient Self-Determination Act specifies that all institutionalized adults receiving medical care from federal funding (Medicaid or Medicare) be given information on their legal rights under state law to accept or refute medical/surgical treatment and the right to formulate advance directives. A signed advance directive, or lack thereof, must be documented in the medical record.[47]

Inherent in any consideration of informed consent is the concept of an individual's constitutional right to privacy, which includes the right to be left alone and not invaded or treated against his/her will. This includes insertion of all feeding tubes, including those nonsurgically implanted.[7] Although generally not an issue with terminally ill adults, the patient's ethical and legal right of self-determination as guaranteed by the informed consent doctrine is not absolute. The state may exert its power to limit the right of personal liberty on the basis of several concepts: (a) the preservation of life, (b) the prevention of suicide, (c) the protection of innocent third parties (especially the financial and emotional interests of minor children), and (d) the protection of the ethical integrity and professional discretion of the medical profession.[3,9,47]

Patients are either decisionally "competent" or "incompetent." Adults are presumed to be legally competent whether or not they have been diagnosed as terminally ill and are thus theoretically capable of participating in defining parameters of medical treatment for themselves. Otherwise, a formal court declaration of "incompetence" is required for this purpose. When a patient's competence is challenged, examination and testimony by a psychiatrist or psychologist are required. The issue generally arises when the patient and medical staff disagree on the use of life-sustaining treatments.[3,7-9,11,13,48-51]

COMPETENT PATIENT

Theoretically, the competent patient has the legal right to refuse all oral food, as well as any mechanical delivery of nutrients. On the other hand, the patient has the theoretical option to choose from the available modalities of nutrition support that may include an invasive, technically sophisticated medical procedure, such as total parenteral nutrition (TPN), even if hydration and nutrients would prolong the intractable pain of the dying process. The appropriate designation of "do not resuscitate" status does not automatically preclude other aggressive medical intervention, such as parenteral nutrition, if that is what the patient needs and desires, and it is available.[3]

The legal resolution of two cases illustrates the issues the courts must consider. A New York State Supreme Court justice ruled in February 1984 that an 85-year-old retired college president, who was alert but depressed, had the right to refuse to eat and to refuse surgery that would allow him to be fed artificially.[38] Although the patient was confined to a wheelchair and had a variety of cardiovascular diseases, his condition was not imminently life-threatening. The decision not to eat was made with the consent of the man's family and his court-appointed guardian. The man died after a 45-day fast.

Beverly Requena, a competent 55-year-old hospital patient with amyotropic lateral sclerosis (ALS), was completely paralyzed from the neck down. On April 4, 1985, she agreed to be placed on a respirator. At that time she had limited ability to suck in fluids through a straw. That ability was deteriorating rapidly and there were significant nutritional deficits, such as an 18-lb weight loss in 2 weeks. Her ability to make sounds was lost in May 1986, although she still maintained the ability to form words with her lips. Communication was also accomplished by eye-blinking responses to questions and by an alphabet board and computer.

Approximately a year and a half after admission to a New Jersey hospital, she informed the hospital that when she did lose her ability to swallow, she did not want to be fed by a tube. Subsequent to Requena's admission the hospital had instituted a policy against withholding or withdrawing artificial feeding or fluids. Arrangements for her transfer to another facility were suggested. Requena refused to consent to a transfer because she had come to like the hospital and had a good relationship with her caregivers. The hospital therefore sought a court order to compel her to leave. The court, in an order almost immediately affirmed on appeal, denied the hospital's request, ruling that a transfer would subject her to emotional and psychological harm, and that the interest of the hospital staff had to be subordinated to the interest of the patient in this case, given that the patient was not asking the hospital staff to do anything, but rather to refrain from taking actions against her will.[52]

INCOMPETENT PATIENTS

Attempting to establish the preferences for treatment or nontreatment of the legally "incompetent" patient is a complicated and often perplexing process. There are several methods for attempting to surmise what the patient would have wanted under the present medical circumstances. First, the patient may have told family members how much or how little use of mechanical means he or she endorses to delay the moment of death.

There are cases in New Jersey and Massachusetts[37,43,45,53] that support the right of self-determination as verbally expressed to family members, friends, and health care professionals which include discontinuing a feeding tube for the nonterminally ill patient who is in a persistent vegetative state. With proper nutrition and nursing care, PVS patients such as Karen Ann Quinlan can live many years without any hope of regaining cognitive or physical functioning.[37] The position adopted by the AMA Council on Ethical and Judicial Affairs in 1986 specifies that "it is not unethical to discontinue all means of life prolonging treatment, including nutrition or hydration, for the PVS patient."[6] Although ADA's position addresses the terminally ill rather than the PVS category of incompetent patients, it will refer to PVS cases for the purpose of discussion.

Another method of attempting to surmise what the patient would have wanted includes a written document such as a "living will" or "durable power of attorney for health care," which directs a range of life-sustaining procedures to be withheld, withdrawn, or continued according to the wishes of the individual. Although helpful when available, such materials are not without their problems. They may have different legal effects in different states. In addition, tube feeding and TPN may not be addressed specifically and some states exclude fluids and nutrition as interventions that can be refused through the living will mechanism.[3,7,9]

In a Florida Supreme Court decision, the court ruled in favor of Helen Corbett, a terminally ill patient who had been in a persistent vegetative state for 3 years.[41] The higher court overturned an earlier decision that prohibited the removal of the nasogastric tube, concluding that the patient maintained her right to refuse artificial feeding, a right that extends even to persons who are not able to act on their own behalf. In this case, as in others, what is of utmost importance is to attempt to ascertain what the patient would have wanted and to act in his or her best interests. The court concluded that patients could exercise their rights to refuse fluids and nutrition by means other than using a living will document.

Nejdl-Barber case. An example of the conflict that can result when trying to choose between two difficult alternatives is evidenced in the murder charges that were brought against two California physicians, Robert Nejdl and Neil Barber. The physicians decided to withdraw intravenous nutrition and hydration from a postoperative anoxia patient who had been in a coma for 5 days.[42] Fifty-five-year-old Clarence Herbert had undergone an ileostomy closure, a simple surgical procedure. In the recovery room, he suffered a cardiorespiratory arrest, which caused severe brain damage. The patient's wife was informed that her husband was "brain dead," and permission was granted for the removal of all machines. The patient died from dehydration and pneumonia 1 week after the intravenous nutrition and hydration tubes were disconnected.

At a preliminary hearing on March 9, 1983, the presiding judge of the California Court of Appeals dismissed the criminal charges against Nejdl and Barber because there was no evidence of malicious intent. Perhaps the most significant aspect of the ruling [42] that is pertinent to this discussion stated that:

> Medical nutrition and hydration may not always provide net benefits to patients. Medical procedures to provide nutrition and hydration are more similar to other medical procedures than to typical human ways of providing nutrition and hydration. Their benefits and burdens ought to be evaluated in the same manner as other medical procedures.

It should be noted that although Herbert was neither terminally ill nor brain dead, the court approved the withdrawal of intravenous nutrition and hydration. The prognosis for return to cognitive functioning was considered hopeless. The court indicated that there was no medical or legal obligation to continue treatment once it has proved to be ineffective.

Conroy case. A landmark decision rendered by the New Jersey Supreme Court in January 1985 found no distinction between a feeding tube and a respirator in determining whether to withdraw life-sustaining care for a competent or incompetent patient with a limited life expectancy, "provided that is what the patient wants or would want."[43]

Claire C. Conroy had severe organic brain syndrome and was unable to speak but responded to noxious or painful stimuli by moaning. She was neither mentally competent nor comatose. Although she was not categorized as terminally ill, there were differences of medical opinion as to whether she had a life expectancy of less than a year. She lay in a fetal position, and was fed through a nasogastric tube. Physical diagnoses included arteriosclerotic heart disease, hypertension, and diabetes mellitus, which contributed to necrotic gangrenous ulcers on her left foot. In 1983, two orthopedic surgeons recommended that Conroy's foot be amputated in order to save her life. Her guardian, a nephew, refused consent for the surgery. Contrary to medical predictions, Conroy did not die from the gangrene.

The guardian then petitioned the court to have her feeding tube discontinued. Pertinent social history indicated that the patient had never married and had few friends and that her nephew guardian was the sole remaining relative. He had maintained a close relationship with Conroy over 50 years and visited her often. There was no conflict of interest over inheritance. The nephew testified that the patient "feared and avoided doctors and that to the best of his knowledge, she had never visited a doctor until she became incompetent in 1979." The lower court denied the petition, and concluded that "withdrawal of the nasogastric tube would be tantamount to killing her—not simply letting her die—and that such active euthanasia was ethically impermissible."

The case was then appealed to a higher court. On February 15, 1983, the patient died of natural causes with the feeding tube in place. Even though Conroy's death made the case moot, the petition was taken to the New Jersey Supreme Court because the future implications for other cases were so important.[22,54] The resulting landmark decision,[44] rendered almost 2 years after her death, clearly specified that it was her autonomy, not her life expectancy, which was at issue.

It should be noted that if she was competent, Conroy's right to self-determination would not be affected by her medical condition or prognosis; a young, generally healthy person, if competent, has the same right to decline life-saving treatment as a competent elderly person who is terminally ill.

Mary O'Connor case. Mary O'Connor had suffered a series of strokes making her "severely demented" and "profoundly incapacitated"; she was paralyzed but could feel pain. She was able to minimally communicate, but was mentally incompetent to make a medical decision. Her two daughters refused to agree to have a nasogastric tube inserted to prolong her life, based on the previous statements made by their mother. The hospital sought a court order to have the tube placed, and both the trial court and intermediate appeals court refused on the grounds that there was clear and convincing evidence that O'Connor would not have wanted the tube inserted. Nonetheless, New York's highest court reversed the decision and ordered the tube inserted.

The court concluded that even though O'Connor had consistently expressed her wishes not to have her life prolonged by "artificial means" or to "lose her dignity" and that it was "monstrous to keep someone alive...by using machinery and things like that when they were not going to get better," that she never specifically said she would not want to be tube fed. The court also rejected the substituted judgment doctrine, saying only the patient herself, not the patient's family, could make a determination to refuse life-sustaining treatment.

Until this case is modified by legislation, the only effective way New York citizens can refuse life-sustaining medical treatment after they become incompetent is to sign a durable power of attorney in which they designate another person (usually a friend or relative they know well and trust) to set limits on treatment decisions made for them. The court specifically found such a document legally effective to permit the individual designated in it to refuse medical treatment, including tube feeding.[40]

Table 4.1

General Considerations Regarding Nutrition Care For The Terminally Ill Adult

I. Each case is unique and must be handled individually.

II. The patient's expressed desire for extent of medical care is a primary guide for determining the level of nutrition intervention.

III. The expected benefits, in contrast to the potential burdens, of non-oral feeding must be evaluated by the health care team and discussed with the patient. The focus of care should emphasize patient physical and psychological comfort.

IV. The decision to forgo hydration or nutrition support should be weighed carefully because such a decision may be difficult or impossible to reverse within a period of days or weeks.

V. The decision to forgo "heroic" medical treatment does not preclude baseline nutrition support.

VI. The physician's written diet order in the medical chart documents the decision to administer or forgo nutrition support. The dietitian should participate in this decision.

VII. The institution's ethics committee, if available, should assist in establishing and implementing defined, written guidelines for nutrition support protocol. The dietitian should be a required member of or consultant to such a committee.

Nancy Cruzan case. On January 11, 1983, Nancy Cruzan, then age 25, lost control of her automobile and lost consciousness when she was thrown into a ditch. Cardiopulmonary resuscitation was performed for approximately 12 to 14 minutes at the site of the accident. She was transferred to a hospital and diagnosed as having a lacerated liver and coma secondary to anoxia. She did not respond to rehabilitative programs and remained in a persistent vegetative state. She was not brain dead and therefore didn't require a respirator to breathe. A gastrostomy tube had been surgically inserted approximately 1 month after her accident.

For 5 years Cruzan's parents drove 90 miles a week to visit her. Then, after agonizing deliberation and with the counseling of religious, medical, and legal experts, they requested that the hospital remove the feeding tube. They strongly believed that their daughter would not want to live indefinitely in a "locked up" existence as a human "vegetable." When the request was refused by hospital medical administration, they petitioned the court on March 9, 1988, to seek judicial sanction for their request.

The trial court, the lowest court in Missouri, concluded from the testimony presented by Cruzan's parents, sister, and a close friend that her conversations shortly before the accident strongly suggested that she would not want to indefinitely exist in a persistent vegetative state. Permission was granted to remove the feeding tube.[53] This judicial decision was consistent with the prevailing national trend of other court cases involving PVS patients on feeding tubes who had not left written directives but had discussed their preferences not to be sustained as a human vegetable.

The lower court's decision was immediately appealed and action was suspended to remove the feeding tube. The Missouri Supreme Court reversed the lower court's decision and denied permission to remove the feeding tube from an incompetent patient who had not left a written expression of her wishes to discontinue all treatment, including artificial feeding. The court disregarded the testimony given by the family, as well as the recommendation of the court-appointed guardian, who said it was in Cruzan's best interest to discontinue tube feeding. The court held that this was not "clear and convincing evidence" because it was inherently unreliable. The Missouri Supreme Court said that the state's interest was not in the "quality" of life but in the preservation of life, no matter how severely diminished the quality of life.[53]

The US Supreme Court granted certiorrari to hear the Cruzan case as the first case regarding right to refuse life-sustaining treatment. The question was whether Missouri had violated Nancy Cruzan's constitutional rights by not requiring the hospital to withdraw life-sustaining treatment, the feeding tube, under the specific circumstances. On June 25, 1990, in a close vote of 5 to 4, the US Supreme Court affirmed the state of Missouri's discretion to impose a very strict standard for "clear and convincing" evidence.[5] Each state may set its own standard of what "clear and convincing" means. Courts may be uncomfortable accepting oral substituted judgment unsupported by written evidence of what the patient would have chosen.

The significant implications of the Cruzan case are:

- there is a protected right to refuse life-sustaining treatment, including tube feeding;
- state statutes that distinguish nutrition support from other "medical treatment" may be unconstitutional;
- states may require a strict "clear and convincing" evidence standard for noncompetent patients, who have not left a written directive of their preferences. This emphasizes the need for written directives, such as health care proxies.

On August 30, 1990, papers were filed that presented three new witnesses who testified that Cruzan would not want continued life-sustaining medical treatment. Several months later, the State of Missouri withdrew from the case. This meant that no remaining party to the case objected to the removal of the tube. Judge Charles E. Teel, Jr, of the Jasper County Courthouse granted permission to remove the feeding tube on December 14, 1990.[45] Cruzan's feeding tube was removed, and her family maintained a vigil until she died, 12 days later.[55]

Conclusion. In the past few years, some of the pressing legal questions on the sensitive area of forgoing medical treatment have begun to be answered. Much remains to be clarified. However, the cases have established some general guidelines.

Courts have recognized that decisionally capable adults have the right to refuse treatment, including artificial feeding.[56] This right is not conditional on the prognosis. This right to self-determination and control over medical decisions is protected by the due process clause of the 14th Amendment of the US Constitution.[5] In the case of incompetent adults, caretakers and family should first try to ascertain the patient's wishes. What "clear and convincing evidence" of a patient's desired wishes includes is unclear. More cases are needed to "define the clear and convincing standard in an operational manner."[14] The use of advance directives and patient-appointed surrogates will help.[47] If those wishes can be dependably ascertained, they should be followed. If they cannot be ascertained, a decision must be made in accordance with the patient's "best interests." A national standard of practice on who should be the best surrogate for the patient is needed.[14]

To protect the patient, the professional, and the facility, there must be a mutual understanding of the local law governing the specific circumstances of the case. Misinformation abounds, but ignorance is no excuse for failing to follow the law. Seeking legal counsel is an integral part of operating within this framework.

MEDICAL CONSIDERATIONS

Generally, compassionate palliative care becomes the fundamental, realistic medical goal in caring for the terminally ill adult. Each patient is unique, and care should be constantly reassessed for each individual. The focus of palliative care is directed toward lessening the pain, psychological distress, and symptoms without actually attempting to cure.

The continuous assessment of the wide spectrum of symptoms is necessary. Amelioration of problems such as nausea, vomiting, insomnia, and anxiety is a common objective. Emotional comfort and support should be provided continuously by the health care staff to both patient and family, through verbal and nonverbal communication.

Table 4.2

Considerations for Examining the Efficacy of Providing Aggressive Nutrition Support

I.   Will nutrient support, either oral or mechanical, improve the patient's quality of life during the final stages of morbidity by increasing physical strength or resistance to infections?

II. Will nutrient support, either oral or mechanical, provide the following to the patient: emotional comfort, decreased anxiety about disease cachexia, improved self-esteem with cosmetic benefits, improved interpersonal relationships, or relief from the fear of abandonment?

III. Oral feedings are the preferred choice. Tube feeding is generally the next logical step. Parenteral nutrition should be considered only when other routes are impossible or inadequate to meet the comfort needs of the patient.

IV. Oral intake

A. Oral feeding should be advocated whenever possible. Food and control of food intake may give comfort and pleasure. The most important priority is to provide food according to the patient's individual wishes.

B. Efforts should be made to enhance the patient's physical and emotional enjoyment of food by encouraging staff and family assistance in feeding the debilitated patient.

C. Nutrition supplements, including commercial products and other alternatives, should be used to encourage intake and ameliorate symptoms associated with hunger, thirst, or malnutrition.

D. The therapeutic rationale of previous diet prescriptions for an individual patient should be reevaluated. Many dietary restrictions can be liberalized. Coordination of medication or medication schedules with the diet should be discussed with the physician, with the objective of maximizing food choice and intake by the patient.

E. The patient's right to self-determination must be considered in determining whether to allow the patient to consume foods that are not generally permitted within the diet prescription.

V. Tube feeding or parenteral feeding
    A. Palliative care is the usual realistic goal. However, a palliative care plan does not automatically preclude aggressive nutrition support.
    B. Facilities should provide and distribute written protocols for the provision of and termination of tube feedings and parenteral feedings. The protocols should be reviewed periodically, and revised if necessary, by the health care team. Legal and ethical counsel should be routinely sought during the development and interpretation of the guidelines.
    C. The patient's informed preference for the level of nutrition intervention is paramount. The patient or guardian should be advised on how to accomplish feeding if the patient wants maximal nutrition care.
    D. Feeding may not be desirable if death is expected within hours or a few days and the effects of partial dehydration or the withdrawal of nutrition support will not adversely alter patient comfort.
    E. Potential benefits vs burdens of tube feeding or parenteral feeding should be weighed on the basis of specific facts concerning the patient's medical and mental status, as well as on facility options and limitations.

Food and drink have both psychological and physical functions that may play very special and sometimes central roles in the care of the terminally ill person. Food has strong emotional and symbolic overtones that include maternal nurturing, as well as religious, cultural, and social values.[25] For the patient able to accept and perhaps enjoy oral intake, previous dietary restrictions should be minimized or eliminated, depending on the potential consequences. The dietitian should work closely with the physician and nurse to coordinate administration of pain medication to maximize enjoyment of food. The actual or illusory source of strength, nurturing, comfort, and caring provided by food should be encouraged. Family interaction and socialization, especially at mealtime, should also be encouraged.

Does good medical practice require the provision of food and water for all patients? There is increasing professional opinion that there are circumstances in which feeding by any means becomes a monumental and futile task. Sometimes the risks, burdens of pain, and discomfort of providing nutrition support substantially outweigh the benefits.[6,20-24] For the individual case in which there is extreme medical deterioration, without a reasonable possibility of remediation, nutrition support may be medically contraindicated. Nutrition intervention may be determined to be futile treatment that exacerbates the distress of dying. Objective medical assessment of the patient's status in relation to the potential medical complications of each modality of feeding and hydration needs careful scrutiny and documentation. (See "Nutrition considerations.")

Are dehydration and starvation painful? For those who have sensation of thirst and hunger, there may be varying degrees of discomfort.[57,58] Do individuals in a coma retain those sensations? Clinicians and researchers are only beginning to explore this topic.[25] Such sensations depend on many variables, including the patient's specific pathological condition(s), the level and kind of pain medication, the mental alertness of the patient, and the environment in which the patient is receiving care. Each of those variables may have bearing on the course of action taken and should be weighed individually when a decision about nutrition support is pending. It is also important to consider that it could take weeks or even months to reverse starvation or semistarvation.[57,58]

Each patient presents with a unique combination of medical problems. Peripheral veins may be in such a deteriorated condition as not to permit intravenous hydration or nutrition support. Aspirational pneumonia or diarrhea may have proved to be real problems with enteral tube feeding. Intestinal obstruction or fistulas may suggest central vein nutrition support, but the latter may be too invasive or expensive or require a specialized team that is not available.

Because the effects of dehydration are frequently a more urgent factor than the effects of inadequate or no food, a review of techniques that may provide comfort is germane. Nurses use ice chips or glycerin swabbing of the mouth to relieve the thirst of patients unable to consume fluids. Dry mouth may be a side effect of medications or the disease and not necessarily a signal of the hydration status. Moreover, hospice workers have reported some potentially beneficial effects of dehydration[23]:

- Dehydration can reduce the patient's secretions and excretions, thus decreasing breathing problems, vomiting, and incontinence.
- Dehydration usually leads to death through hemoconcentration and hyperosmolality with subsequent azotemia, hypernatremia, and hypercalcemia—all of which produce a sedative effect on the brain just before death.

    In most cases, the nutrition goals for the terminally ill adult is not based on the parameters of nitrogen balance and desired weight as used with the nonterminally ill population. The subject is perplexing, and there is no current consensus on what is appropriate. Nutrition support decisions—like all health care decisions—may be based on less than perfect information and an intent to act in the patient's best interests.

NUTRITION CONSIDERATIONS

Helping the physician and the terminally ill patient weigh the potential benefits against the burdens of the various nutrition alternatives is a challenging and complex task. Health care professionals and patients must learn to cope with the stress that results from the fact that much uncertainty accompanies each illness.[59]

CRITERIA FOR DETERMINING APPROPRIATE LEVELS OF NUTRITION CARE

When developing the nutrition care plan for the terminally ill adult, the dietitian needs to consider three essential criteria:

1. The patient's medical status as diagnosed and documented by the physician(s).[1-4] This is an ongoing reassessment process. Continuous good communication among the interdisciplinary health care team members, as well as with the patient and family, is essential.[5]

2. The patient's informed preference[8,9,13,60] for which level of nutrition support is desired during the various stages of dying. The dietitian should show utmost sensitivity to the patient's wishes. This, too, is an ongoing reassessment and interaction process.

3. The ethical and legal framework within which feeding alternatives are considered and policies formulated. Health care practitioners, lawyers, legislators, theologians, and human rights advocate groups,[61,62] as well as the general public, are generating much debate on this topic. The problems of our society are constantly changing; what is acceptable protocol today may be obsolete tomorrow.

The basic process used to develop the nutrition care plan for the terminally ill patient is similar to that recommended for the critically ill patient.[63] The primary difference is that information will usually be evaluated from an orientation of palliation rather than cure.

Table 4.3

Considerations for Examining the Efficacy of Forgoing or Discontinuing Aggressive Nutrition Support

I. Questions that can help to determine the potential burdens include:
   A. What is the level of risk for potential medical and metabolic complications from each available nutrition alternative?
   B. Will the administration of tube feeding or total parenteral nutrition at home or in a health care facility be contraindicated because of staffing, monitoring ability, or financial constraints?
   C. Will the nutritional benefits of the insertion of an enteral or parenteral feeding tube during hospitalization create feelings of abandonment if tube feeding is unavailable upon discharge?

II. Forgoing or discontinuing enteral or parenteral nutrition support may be considered when some or all of the following are present:
   A. Death is imminent, within hours or a few days.
   B. Enteral or parenteral feeding will probably worsen the condition, symptoms, or pain, such as during shock, when

pulmonary edema or diarrhea, vomiting, or aspiration would cause further complications.

C. A competent patient has expressed an informed preference not to receive aggressive nutrition support that would be ineffective in improving the quality of life and/or which may be perceived by the patient as undignified, degrading, and physically or emotionally unacceptable.

D. If available and legally recognized, written advanced directives such as the "living will" or "durable power of attorney for medical care" may indicate the preference of an incompetent patient. Otherwise, the next of kin or patient appointed surrogate of an incompetent patient should be consulted about the patient's probable preference for the level of nutrition intervention, as well as state law.

III. Written ethical guidelines for assessing and implementing these considerations should be established through the facility's ethics committee, if available, and in accordance with legal guidance.

IV. Legal precedents and regulations or statutes establishing feeding parameters within local and state jurisdiction should be considered when deciding to require or forgo nutrition support. The facility's written protocol and legal counsel should also be consulted.

First, the dietitian reviews the nutritionally relevant objective data. If available, the physician's prognosis for life expectancy is crucial, although somewhat limited in precision. Other data to be examined include medical diagnosis; findings from a physical examination, such as symptoms and sources of discomfort; and previous treatments, including modified diets and medications.[63] Current status may be difficult to confirm if diagnostic testing has been discontinued in accordance with patient comfort goals. Nursing or social service chart notes may include the patient's religious, philosophical, social, emotional, and financial concerns that affect dying.[64]

The second source of information is subjective data collected by the dietitian upon visiting the patient. What is the potential ability of the patient to ingest food? Factors to be assessed include consciousness, dysphagia, severity of vomiting and nausea, and degree of discomfort and pain.[63] Is the patient explicitly indicating which level of nutrition care is currently preferred? The patient may be requesting special food that is not ordinarily available in a hospital. On the other hand, the patient may be adamantly rejecting all food. Respect for the patient's right to refuse food and fluid can cause serious harm to the patient; therefore, the health care provider needs to explore the patient's reason for refusing food and fluid. The health care provider should establish that the competent patient accurately understands the situation, the choices available, and the benefit and harm of each choice. Indications for the withholding of food and fluid include feeding being futile or harmful. However, in most cases, food and fluid are in the best interest of the patient, whether they provide nourishment or comfort.[61]

From the objective and subjective data, the dietitian can develop a nutrition care plan.[60] This stage of the analysis and formulation relies heavily upon the dietitian's expertise in integrating the scientific basis of applied human nutrition in health and disease.[65,66] Justification of the recommendations should be documented in a clear, concise, logical presentation, using as many concrete data as are available. Recommendations may need to be supported with authoritative references that reinforce credibility. For example, the use of statistics from published research or from data collected with the individual institution provides a quantitative means of weighing the strengths and weaknesses of each nutrition modality. However, statistics should also be used with caution. Technical expertise as well as value judgments influence the interpretation of objective data.

During the next step, the collaborative decision-making process, sufficient information should be presented in a clear, unbiased manner to the patient or surrogate decision maker by the physician and dietitian to facilitate an informed decision.[12] The nutrition care plan will reflect choices agreed upon during this process. Follow-up and continuous reassessment of the effectiveness and desirability of the care plan are mandatory and should be documented in the medical chart accordingly. Continued discussion with the patient and health care team members is also required to ensure effective coordination of care.

The dietitian must be flexible in attempting to meet the nutrition needs of each dying patient. Dietitians are appropriate participants in such bioethical decisions.[2,67,68] Emphasizing the art of providing emotional support—TLC (tender loving care)—may be a more useful guide than concentrating on the science of providing RDAs (Recommended Daily Allowances) in meeting the patient's multiple needs for food.

References

1. Ad Hoc Committee on Medical Ethics, American College of Physicians. American College of Physicians Ethical Manual: Part II. Research: Other ethical issues. Recommended reading. *Ann Intern Med.* 1984;101:263–274.
2. Gallagher-Allred CR. *Nutritional Care of the Terminally Ill.* Gaithersburg, Md: Aspen Publishers; 1989.
3. President's Commission for the Study of Ethical Problems in Medicine and Biomedical and Behavioral Research. *Deciding to Forego Life Sustaining Treatment.* Washington, DC: US Government Printing Office; 1983. 83-600503.
4. Wanzer SH, Adelstein SJ, Cranford RE, Federman DD, Hook ED, Moertel CG, Safar P, Stone A, Taussig HB, van Eys J. The physician's responsibility toward hopelessly ill patients. *N Engl J Med.* 1984:310:955–959.
5. Nancy Beth Cruzan, by her parents and Co-Guardians, Lester L. Cruzan, et ux, Petitioners v. Director, Missouri Department of Health, et al. Supreme Court Docket Number 88-1503. Argued: December 6, 1989; Decided: June 25, 1990.
6. *Statement of the Council on Ethical and Judicial Affairs: Withholding or Withdrawing Life Prolonging Medical Treatment.* Chicago, Ill: American Medical Association; 1986.

7. *Guidelines on the Termination of Life-Sustaining Treatment and the Care of the Dying. A Report by the Hastings Center.* Briarcliff Manor, NY: Hastings Center; 1987.

8. President's Commission for the Study of Ethical Problems in Medicine and Biomedical and Behavioral Research. *Making Health Care Decisions: The Ethical and Legal Implications of Informed Consent in the Patient/Practitioner Relationship.* Vols 1–3. Washington, DC: US Government Printing Office; 1982. 82:6000637.

9. Robertson JA. *The Rights of the Critically Ill: An American Civil Liberties Union Handbook.* New York, NY: Bantam Books; 1983.

10. Beauchamp TL, Childress JF. *Principles of Biomedical Ethics.* 2nd ed. New York, NY: Oxford University Press; 1983.

11. Special Committee on Biomedical Ethics. *Values in Conflict.* Chicago, Ill: American Hospital Association; 1985.

12. Code of Ethics for the Profession of Dietetics. *J Am Diet Assoc.* 1988; 88:1592–1593.

13. Paris J, McCormick R. *The Catholic Tradition on the Use of Nutrition and Fluids.* America, 356-361, May 2, 1987.

14. Lo B, Steinbrook R. Beyond the Cruzan case: the U.S. Supreme Court and medical practice. *Ann Intern Med.* 1991;114:895–901.

15. Jonsen AR, Siegler M, Winslade WJ. *Clinical Ethics.* New York, NY: Macmillan Publishing Co; 1982.

16. Purtilo RB, Cassel CK. *Ethical Dimensions in the Health Professions.* Philadelphia, Pa: WB Saunders Co; 1981.

17. Reich WT, ed. *Encyclopedia of Bioethics.* Vols 1, 2. New York, NY: Free Press; 1978.

18. Thompson JB, Thompson HO. *Ethics in Nursing.* New York, NY: Macmillan Publishing Co; 1981.

19. Boisaubin EV. Ethical issues in the nutritional support of the terminal patient. *J Am Diet Assoc.* 1984;84:529–531.

20. Curran WJ. Defining appropriate medical care: providing nutrients and hydration for the dying. *N Engl J Med.* 1985;313:940–942.

21. Cohen EN Cohen MM. Artificial feeding and patient's rights: recent developments and recommendations. *Med Staff Counselor.* 1988;2(3):23.

22. Dresser R. Discontinuing nutrition support: a review of the case law. *J Am Diet Assoc.* 1985;85:1289–1292.

23. Dresser RS, Boisaubin EV. Ethics, law and nutrition support. *Arch Intern Med.* 1985;145:122–124.

24. Lynn J. *By No Extraordinary Means.* Bloomington, Ind: Indiana University Press; 1986.

25. Mishkin B. Withholding and withdrawing nutrition support: advance planning for hard choices. *Nutr Clin Pract.* 1986;1:50–52.

26. Micetich DC, Steinecker PH, Thomasma DC. Are intravenous fluids morally required for a dying patient? *Arch Intern Med.* 1983;143:975–978.

27. Ott DB. Hospice care: an opportunity for dietetic services. *J Am Diet Assoc.* 1985;85:223–225.

28. Zerwech J. The dehydration question. *Nursing.* 1983;13:17–19.

29. Rango N. The nursing home resident with dementia: clinical care, ethics, and policy implications. *Ann Intern Med.* 1985;102:836–841.

30. Kubler-Ross E, Warshaw M. *To Live Until We Say Good-Bye.* Englewood Cliffs, NJ: Prentice-Hall; 1978.

31. Steinbrook R, Lo B, Tirpack J, Dilley J, Volberding P. Ethical dilemmas in caring for patients with the acquired immunodeficiency syndrome. *Ann Intern Med.* 1985;103:787–790.

32. Olick RS. Brain death, religious freedom, public policy: NJs landmark legislative initiative. *Kennedy Institute of Ethics J.* 1991;1(4):675.

33. Epstein C. *Nursing the Dying Patient.* Englewood Cliffs, NJ: Prentice-Hall; 1975.

34. *Hospice Standards Manual.* Chicago, Ill: Joint Commission on Accreditation of Hospitals; 1986

35. *Matter of Earle Spring,* 380 Mass 629, 405 NE2d 115 (1980).

36. *Matter of Shirley Dinnerstein,* 380 NE2d 134 (Mass. App. 1978).

37. *Matter of Karen Ann Quinlan,* 70 NJ 10, 335 A2d 647 (1976).

38. *In the Matter of the Application of Plaza Health and Rehabilitation Center.* (New York Supreme Court, Syracuse, February 6, 1984, Miller, J.).

39. *Bouvia v Superior Court of the State of California for the County of Los Angeles,* No. B 019134, Super Ct C583828, filed April 16, 1986, p. 20.

40. *In regarding Westchester County, Medical Center (Mary O'Connor)* 72 NY2d 517, 534 NYC2d 886, 531 NE2d 607, 1988.

41. *Corbett v The Honorable Joseph P. D'Alessandro, District Court of Appeal of Florida,* No. 85-1052, filed April 18, 1986.

42. *Barber and Nejdl v Superior Court of State of California,* 147 Cal App3d 1006, 195 Cal Reptr 484 (1983).

43. *Matter of Claire C. Conroy,* 190 NJ Super 453, 464 A2d 303 (1983).

44. *In re Conroy,* 486 A2d 1209 (NJ 1985).

45. *Cruzan v Mouton.* Missouri Circuit Court, Jasper County, Probate Division at Carthage, Estate No. CV384-9P, Dec 14, 1990.

46. Butterworth CW, Blackburn GL. Hospital malnutrition. *Nutr Today.* 1975;10:18.

47. LaPuma J, Orentilicher D, Moss RJ. Advance Directives on Admission. Clinical Implications and Analysis of the Patient Self Determination Act of 1990. *JAMA.* 1991;266:402-405.

48. Annas GJ, Densberger JE. Competence to refuse medical treatment: Autonomy vs. paternalism. *Toledo Law Rev.* 1984;15:561-595.

49. Bullough B. *The Law & The Expanding Nursing Role.* New York, NY: Appleton-Century-Crofts; 1980.

50. Louisell DW, Williams H. *Medical Malpractice.* New York, NY: Matthew Bender; 1990.

51. Reidy EB, Reidy DE. Malpractice law and the dietitian. *J Am Diet Assoc.* 1975;67:335-338.

52. *Beverly Requena—Matter of Beverly Requena,* 213 NJ Super 475, 517 A 2 886 (1986).

53. *Cruzan v Harmon,* 760 SW2d 408 (Mo Banc, 1988).

54. Bursztajn H. *Medical Choices/Medical Chances.* New York, NY: Routhledge; 1990.

55. Belkin L. "Missouri Seeks to Quit Case of Comatose Patient." *NY Times.* October 12, 1990, p A15.

56. Annas GJ. Do feeding tubes have more rights than patients? *Hastings Cent Rep.* 1986;16:26-28.

57. Winick M. *Hunger Disease: Studies by the Jewish Physicians in the Warsaw Ghetto.* New York, NY: John Wiley & Sons; 1979.

58. Young VR, Scrimshaw ND. The physiology of starvation. *Sci Am.* 1971;225:14-21.

59. Cassem N. Treatment decisions in irreversible illness. In: Cassem N, Hackett T, eds. *MGH Handbook of General Hospital Psychiatry.* St Louis, Mo: CV Mosby; 1978.

60. *New role delineation. Role Delineation Study: Technical Report.* Chicago, Ill: American Dietetic Association; 1989.

61. *Guidelines on Withdrawing or Withholding Food and Fluids. Ethics in Nursing: Position Statements and Guidelines.* Kansas City, Mo: American Nurses Association; 1988.

62. Nelson LJ. The law, professional responsibility and decisions to forego treatment. *QRB*. 1986;12:8.
63. Quality Assurance Committee, Dietitians in Critical Care Dietetic Practice Group. *Suggested Guidelines for Nutrition Management of the Critically Ill Patient.* Chicago, Ill: American Dietetic Association; 1984.
64. Perkins HS, Jonsen AR. Dying right in theory and practice: what do we really know of terminal care? *Arch Intern Med*. 1985;145:1460-1463.
65. Shils ME, Young V, eds. *Modern Nutrition in Health and Disease: Dietotherapy.* Philadelphia, Pa: Lea & Febiger; 1988.
66. Rombeau JL, Caldwell MS, eds. *Enteral and Tube Feeding.* Philadelphia, Pa: WB Saunders Co; 1991.
67. Wall MG, Wellman NS, Curry KR, Johnson PM. Feeding the terminally ill: dietitians' attitudes and beliefs. *J Am Diet Assoc*. 1991;91:549-552.
68. Position of The American Dietetic Association: issues in feeding the terminally ill adult. *J Am Diet Assoc*. 1987; 87:78-85.

- ADA Position adopted by the House of Delegates on October 6, 1985, and reaffirmed on October 24, 1991.
- Recognition is given to the following for their contributions:
  Authors: Dorothy G. King, PhD, RD; Julie O'Sullivan Maillet, PhD, RD
  Reviewers: George J. Annas, JD, MPH; Eugene V. Boisaubin, MD; Ronni Chernoff, PhD, RD; John Grant, MD; M. Rosita Schiller, PhD, RD; Robin Spencer Palmisano, JD, RD; Jeanette K. Chambers, PhD, RN; Dietitians in Nutrition Support dietetic practice group; and Gerontological Nutritionists dietetic practice group.
- Approved by the House of Delegates on October 6, 1985, and reaffirmed on October 24, 1991, with updates, to be in effect until November 30, 1996, with an update of cases in 1994. The American Dietetic Association authorizes republication of this Position Paper, in its entirety, provided full and proper credit is given.

5. Continuous Qualtiy Improvement

**Defining the Process
(Transition from QA to CQI)**

**Developing and Implementing a
CQI Plan**

**Sample: Monitoring an Aspect of
Care**

5. Continuous Quality Improvement

Commitment to continuous quality improvement (CQI) must pervade the entire organization. Implementing and maintaining a self-assessment system supports and nurtures CQI in resident care. Ongoing monitoring and evaluation of performance provides caregivers the opportunity for early intervention and/or prevention of potential problems regarding resident care decisions. Appropriate participation of residents in the decisions affecting their care improves the quality of life for all residents served.

Overseeing the provision of optimal nutrition and dietary care to the residents in a nursing facility is the responsibility of the registered dietitian. Implementing and maintaining a CQI program is a proven way of ensuring appropriate nutrition care.

Effective October 1, 1990, an outcome-oriented survey process was mandated in all skilled nursing facilities (SNF) and intermediate care facilities (ICF), now referred to as nursing facilities. This is one of the many changes in long-term care that result from the Omnibus Budget Reconciliation Act (OBRA) of 1987. This new, outcome-oriented survey process is designed to focus on overall quality, resident care, and protection of residents' rights.

Along with a new survey process, OBRA 87 requires the establishment of various committees including safety, utilization review, pharmacy, infection control, and quality assurance. Failure to comply with the new regulations may result in sanctions from Medicaid or Medicare.

The implementation of a facility quality improvement program is necessary to demonstrate deliverance of timely, appropriate, and effective health care. The basic objectives of a CQI program are to identify and aid in correction of quality deficiencies, improve current accepted levels of care, and identify areas of excellent care.

The following excerpt from the *Federal Register* is the new standard mandating quality improvement programs in nursing facilities[1]:

Department of Health and Human Services
Health Care Financing Administration
Quality Assessment and Assurance

Effective October 1, 1990, a facility must maintain a Quality Assessment and Assurance Committee consisting of:

- The director of nursing service;
- A physician designated by the facility; and
- At least three other members of the facility's staff.

The Quality Assessment and Assurance Committee:

- Meets at least quarterly to identify issues with respect to which quality assessment and assurance activities are necessary; and
- Develops and implements appropriate plans of action to correct identified quality deficiencies.

Defining the Process (Transition From QA to CQI)

Historically, quality assurance (QA) was the term used to describe programs designed to assure quality care was being provided. Continuous quality improvement is a concept that is replacing traditional QA philosophies.

Quality improvement is an ongoing process that includes identification of problems or potential risk areas, development of a plan to correct the problem, implementation of a solution, and follow-up to ensure that the problem has been resolved.

The Joint Commission on Accreditation of Health Care Organizations (JCAHO) is a recognized leader in the quality improvement movement in health care facilities. The ten-step process for monitoring and evaluation developed by JCAHO provides a model for setting up a CQI program.

JCAHO'S Ten Steps of Monitoring and Evaluation*

STEP 1: *Assign responsibility.*

Each department director should be responsible for and actively participate in monitoring and evaluation. The director assigns responsibility for the specific duties related to monitoring and evaluation.

STEP 2: *Delineate scope of care.*

Each department director should establish an inventory of its clinical activities. This delineated scope of care provides a basis for identifying those aspects of care that will be the focus of monitoring and evaluation.

STEP 3: *Identify important aspects of care.*

Important aspects of care are those that are high-risk, high-volume, and/or problem-prone. Staff should identify important aspects of care to

---

* From *Hospital Accreditation Survey Program.*[2] Copyright by the Joint Commission on Accreditation of Healthcare Organizations, Oakbrook Terrace, IL. Reprinted with permission.

focus monitoring and evaluation on those areas with the greatest impact on quality of resident care. Examples include evaluation and assessment of residents' nutritional needs, documentation of nutrition assessment and reassessment, and meal service.

STEP 4: *Identify indicators.*

Indicators of quality should be identified for each important aspect of care. An indicator is a well-defined, measurable variable related to the structure, process, or outcome of care. Indicators should be objective and measurable and should help direct attention to potential problems or opportunities to improve care. Indicators should focus on high-volume, high-risk, or problem-prone areas of care. Examples include identification of residents requiring nutrition intervention, timeliness of nutrition assessment and reassessment, and meal satisfaction.

STEP 5: *Establish thresholds for evaluation.*

Thresholds for evaluation are the levels or points at which intensive evaluations of care are triggered. A threshold should be established for each indicator. Thresholds can be based on clinical and quality assurance literature and on the particular experience of the department or organization.

STEP 6: *Collect and organize data.*

Appropriate staff should collect data pertaining to the indicators. Data should be organized to facilitate comparison with the thresholds for evaluation.

STEP 7: *Evaluate care.*

When the cumulative data reach the threshold for evaluation, appropriate staff members should evaluate the care provided to determine whether a problem exists. This evaluation should be sensitive to possible trends and patterns of performance. The evaluation should also attempt to identify causes of any problems or methods by which care or performance may be improved.

STEP 8: *Take actions to improve care and services.*

When problems are identified, action plans should be developed and approved at the appropriate levels and enacted to solve the problem or take the opportunity to improve care.

STEP 9: *Assess the actions and document improvement.*

The effectiveness of those actions should be assessed and documented. If further actions are necessary to solve a problem, they should be taken and their effectiveness assessed.

STEP 10: *Communication of relevant information to the organization-wide quality improvement program.*

Findings from and conclusions of monitoring and evaluation of activities, including actions taken to solve problems and improve care, should be documented and reported through the established channels of communication.

CQI Versus QA

There are major differences between CQI and QA, as shown in *Table 5.1.*

Table 5.1

Differences Between
Continuous Quality Improvement and Quality Assurance

CQI	QA
Evaluates processes and outcomes of care.	Evaluates separate programs.
Improves quality of all services for residents and others.	Ensures quality of resident care.
Focuses on improvement.	Focuses on compliance with JCAHO, state, or federal standards.
Looks at process errors.	Looks at individual errors.
Approach to the program is on continuous improvement, even if no "problem" is identified.	Follows problem-solving approach.
Concurrent studies.	Retrospective studies or audits.
Involves all employees, management, residents, and administration.	Primarily involves management
Breaks down interdepartmental barriers	Focuses on individual departments.
Long-term improvement over time.	Quick fix; usually not permanent.

In summary, CQI reflects a facility's commitment and efforts to improve the overall system. Departments are encouraged to work together to solve problems. The success of this process requires that employees and residents alike be involved in the program. Staff members at all levels of the organization continuously assess and recognize opportunities for change that will improve the quality of resident care.

What About Quality Control?

Quality control is a system or program that measures or monitors day-to-day functions. Examples of dietary quality control activities include monitoring tray assembly speed, refrigerator and freezer temperature control records, dish machine temperature, mechanical condition of equipment, receiving procedures, and chemical storage.

Although these are important areas of concern in all dietary departments, one cannot assume that adequacy in these areas will result in quality nutrition care. Quality control functions will continue to be part of the process of improving delivery of services. The resident-oriented outcomes of CQI are different from quality control. Quality control remains a comparison of day-to-day activities or department functions and established standards.

Areas of care that could directly affect the resident's nutrition status and therefore would be considered CQI activities may include tray accuracy (correct diet as ordered by physician), menu adequacy (daily menu meets Dietary Guidelines food plan), nutritional adequacy of nourishment, timeliness of nutrition intervention, effectiveness of care plan, and/or effectiveness of nutrition therapy.

Developing and Implementing a CQI Plan

The CQI program is a preplanned and systematic process of monitoring and evaluating the quality and appropriateness of care provided. The goal of the program is to improve resident care.

FACILITY PLAN

Before beginning a department CQI program, the facility's overall quality improvement program should be reviewed. The facility's goals for provision of quality care should be reflected in each department's plan. The facility plan includes all departments, employees, and committees. All employees are responsible for understanding their roles in the process of providing CQI to the residents they serve.

DIETARY DEPARTMENT PLAN

Each department is responsible for a plan targeting the services it provides. Participation of all department employees in the planning stages will provide a comprehensive base of information to assess and recognize opportunities for change. Leaders within each department help establish a preplanned, systematic process of monitoring and evaluating the quality and appropriateness of the care provided. Addressing each of the ten steps used in the JCAHO process to organize a department CQI plan is encouraged. Priorities must be set to provide direction to the monitoring and evaluation activities.

ANNUAL CALENDAR OF MONITORING AND EVALUATION

An annual calendar targeting important areas of care to be studied, is helpful for organizing the quality improvement process. Data on problem-prone, high-risk, and high-volume areas of care should be recorded and used in developing an annual plan, as well as for evaluation at the end of the year. The calendar should be used as a tentative guideline and can be changed if more important evaluation needs arise.

FORMAT FOR COMMUNICATING WITH THE QUALITY IMPROVEMENT COMMITTEE AND STAFF

Communications are a cornerstone to successful quality improvement. Reporting the information to the quality improvement committee involves communicating, reporting, and listening. Effective care planning involving the resident and people in many departments depends on communication. Therefore, successful intervention depends on the interaction between individuals and groups. Communication must work at three levels: within the department; between each department and the quality improvement committee; and between departments.

The CQI program is a preplanned and systematic process for monitoring and evaluating the quality and appropriateness of care. When developing a facility or department plan, follow JCAHO's Ten Step guidelines for systematic application.

Sample: Monitoring an Aspect of Care

Monitoring documentation of the nutrition assessment and reassessment is an example of quality improvement that can be conducted by the dietetic technician or dietary manager and the registered dietitian. This aspect of care is considered high volume since a timely nutrition assessment or reassessment is required for all residents in a nursing facility.

Completing an assessment is an initial step in determining and meeting the nutrition needs of the resident. A standard, comprehensive assessment has been established by Health Care Financing Administration (HCFA):

the minimum data set (MDS) for nursing facility resident assessment. The registered dietitian and the dietetic technician or dietary manager are among interdisciplinary personnel who assess the resident on admission. The assessment includes evaluation and documentation of functional status, nutritional status and requirements, psychosocial status, cognitive or mental status, physical condition, clinical findings, skin condition, and drug therapy, plus rehabilitation and discharge potential.

OBRA regulations state that the assessments must be completed within 14 days after the date of admission. State and local interpretive guidelines give specifics on complying with these regulations.

An example of the methodology for monitoring the documentation of nutrition assessment and reassessment is shown in *Table 5.2.*

The next step is to write standards for all areas of documentation. For example:

- *Timeliness of review*: Initial assessment within 14 days of admission. Change of condition within 14 days of condition change. Quarterly reassessment every 3 months and up to 7 days for a revised care plan.
- *Weight*: Current weight in pounds (within 1 month). Reasonable and/or ideal body weight included on initial charts.
- *Weight assessment*: Comparison to reasonable and/or ideal body weight every 6 to 12 months. Assessment of weight gain/loss (including percentage). Ten percent weight loss in 6 months is documented as a significant nutritional risk.
- *Diet order*: Diet order matches physician order. Appropriateness of diet order is assessed in initial evaluation.

After the standards for documentation have been established, a data collection tool should be established. The registered dietitian and dietetic technician or dietary manager decide what information each is responsible for in the charting process. Information is collected for an established period (see example, *Figure 5.1*).

Once data have been collected, the results are evaluated. As noted in Figure 5.1, the threshold for the first indicator is not met. Initial analysis of the data indicates that more charts need to be reviewed to accurately assess the indicator timeliness of nutrition assessment and reassessment.

The second indicator, the completed nutrition assessment or reassessment of the resident, was met only 60% of the time. Review of the data for trends or patterns targets documentation of skin condition, drugs, and bowel program as areas that need improvement.

At this point in the process, an action plan is developed and implemented by the registered dietitian and dietetic technician or dietary manager to correct the problem. The action plan should be monitored and evaluated to ensure that the problem is corrected. Results of the quality improvement study, action, and improvement are reported to the facility's quality improvement committee.

Table 5.2

Aspect of Care:
Documentation of Nutrition Assessment and Reassessment

Indicator	Threshold	Criteria	Data Source	Sample size, Frequency	What is collected from data source	Collected by	Analyzed by
Timeliness of nutrition assessment/ reassessment	95%	Nutrition assessments/ reassessments are completed: Within 14 d of admission Within 14 d of care conferences	Resident* Medical*	All residents for 2 mo; 25% or 20 charts (whichever is greater) may be used if study is conducted retrospectively	Timeliness of nutrition assessment/ reassessment	DT/DM RD	DT/DM RD
Completeness of resident nutrition assessment/ reassessment	90%	The nutrition assessment/ reassessment of the resident is complete.	Resident* Medical record*	All residents for 2 mo; 25% or 20 charts (whichever is greater) may be used if study is conducted retrospectively	The nutrition assessment/ reassessment includes Weight Weight assessment Diet order Food intake Nourishments Hydration status Condition change Signs of malnutrition Lab value Lab value assessment Skin condition Drug interactions Ability to feed self Feeding location Bowel program Goals Plan of care	DT/DM RD	DT/DM RD

*This study may be conducted concurrently or retrospectively.

Printed with permission from Behrens and Blocker.[3]

What If Everything Is Okay?

Occasionally an area of care will be studied and the established threshold will be met. If study of this area of care is to continue the following circumstances should be considered:

- Is this still an important aspect of care? If not, monitoring should stop.
- Is the indicator stated in a way that provides adequate data related to the important aspect of care? If not, the indicator must be developed further to address the important aspect of care adequately.
- Are the sample size and/or frequency of data collection adequate? If not, more frequent monitoring and/or a larger sample should be established.

Figure 5.1

Aspect of Care:
Documentation of Nutrition Assessment and Reassessment

Date: __July 1990__   Criteria Met: Y

Monitored by: __M. Criner, R.D.__   Not Met: N

Chart Reviewed	Brincks, I.	Hackman, L.	Behrens, A.	Hageman, O.	Kruse, B.	Kruse, M.	Linderbaum, E.	Tieskoetter, L.	Wenhake, D.	Beckman, J.	# of Yes	% Criteria/Data met	Threshold
1. Timeliness of Review	Y	Y	Y	Y	Y	Y	Y	Y	Y	N	9/10	90%	95%
2. Weight	Y	Y	N	Y	Y	Y	Y	Y	Y	Y	9/10	90%	
Weight Assessment	Y	Y	N	Y	Y	Y	Y	Y	Y	Y	9/10	90%	
Diet order	Y	Y	Y	Y	Y	Y	Y	Y	Y	Y	10/10	100%	
Food Intake	Y	Y	Y	Y	Y	Y	Y	Y	Y	Y	10/10	100%	
Nourishment Intake	Y	Y	Y	Y	Y	Y	Y	Y	Y	Y	10/10	100%	
Hydration Status	Y	Y	Y	Y	Y	N	Y	Y	Y	Y	9/10	90%	
Change in Condition	Y	Y	Y	Y	Y	Y	Y	Y	Y	Y	10/10	100%	
Physical and clinical signs of malnutrition	Y	Y	Y	Y	Y	Y	Y	Y	Y	Y	10/10	100%	
Lab values	Y	Y	Y	Y	Y	Y	Y	Y	Y	Y	10/10	100%	
Lab value Assessment	Y	Y	Y	Y	Y	Y	Y	Y	Y	Y	10/10	100%	
Skin Condition	Y	Y	Y	Y	Y	N	Y	Y	N	Y	8/10	80%	
Drugs and Interactions	Y	Y	N	Y	Y	Y	N	Y	N	N	6/10	60%	
Ability to Feed Self	Y	Y	Y	Y	Y	N	Y	Y	Y	Y	10/10	100%	
Feeding Location	Y	Y	Y	Y	Y	Y	Y	Y	Y	Y	10/10	100%	
Bowel Program	Y	Y	N	Y	Y	N	Y	Y	Y	N	7/10	70%	
Others	NA										NA	NA	NA
Reassessment of Short and Long Term Goals	Y	Y	Y	Y	Y	N	Y	Y	Y	Y	9/10	90%	
Plan of Care	Y	Y	Y	Y	Y	Y	Y	Y	Y	Y	10/10	100%	
Criteria for completeness met	Y	Y	N	Y	Y	N	Y	Y	N	N	6/10	60%	90%

Note boxes on form:
1. Threshold for Criteria #1 not met–need to review more charts!
2. Threshold for Criteria #2 not met–areas that need improvement are: Skin condition, Drugs, Bowel program

Printed with permission from Behrens and Blocker.[3]

- Would the quality of care improve by decreasing or increasing the threshold? If so, the threshold for evaluation should be changed.
- If the sample size and/or frequency of data collection were decreased, would the quality and appropriateness of the important aspect of care still be conveyed? If so, the sample size and/or frequency can be reduced. If not, they should be maintained at present levels.

Annual Evaluation

An appraisal of the effectiveness of the quality improvement should be completed annually. The purpose of this evaluation is to identify areas of improvement, evaluate the overall effectiveness of the past year's plan, identify changes in each department's scope of service, and develop a monitoring plan for next year.

Guidelines to a Successful CQI Program

- Keep it simple. Do not monitor too many areas of care at once. It's better to solve one problem than to become disillusioned with ten.
- Involve all staff members.
- Encourage (seek) input from residents.
- Focus on improvements and work together. Remember, 85% of all problems are process errors, not people errors.

References

1. Rules and Regulations HCFA. *Federal Register*, Feb 2, 1989; 54:5372.
2. *Hospital Accreditation Survey Preparation. Education Program.* Oak Brook, Ill: Joint Commission on Accreditation of Health Care Organizations; 1991;3:7–13.
3. Behrens RI, Blocker AK. *Making Quality Count.* Ossian, Iowa; Visions for Success; 1990.
4. Behrens RI, Blocker AK. Overview of nutritional assessment. *Consultant Dietitian.* 1991;16:10–11.

6. ASSESSMENT DETERMINANTS

Laboratory Values

Food-Medication Interactions

Enteral and Parenteral Feedings

6. ASSESSMENT DETERMINANTS

Laboratory Values

The nutrition assessment of a resident should include laboratory evaluation. Because the normal range of a value may differ among laboratories, the normal ranges stated by the laboratory that performs the analysis should be used. Laboratory parameters are altered for an elderly resident according to a variety of factors, one of which is nutritional status. Knowledge of what, besides poor nutrition may cause abnormal values fosters accurate assessment. Laboratory values in the elderly resident can be complicated by latent or overt disease, multisystem disease, and physiologic and anatomic changes associated with aging for which normal values have not been determined.[1] Despite the myriad changes, the laboratory values, in conjunction with anthropometric evaluation and diet history information, are valuable.

Prior to assessing laboratory values, the resident's serum osmolality (normal range, 280 to 295 mOsm) should be checked. Hydration status alters laboratory values. Dehydration increases serum osmolality and many other laboratory values; it may cause values to appear high or normal and may mask a deficiency. Overhydration dilutes and lowers the values. Knowing the resident's hydration contributes to a more accurate nutritional diagnosis.

The most useful laboratory values in nutrition assessment are serum albumin, serum transferrin, prealbumin, hematocrit, hemoglobin, glucose, cholesterol, blood urea nitrogen (BUN), and electrolytes, specifically sodium (Na) and potassium (K). If available, creatinine clearance (if renal function is normal) and the total lymphocyte count are also useful. The registered dietitian must be familiar with the reasons for abnormalities besides nutritional status prior to making a judgment. The major causes of abnormalities are listed later in this chapter.

BIOCHEMICAL PARAMETERS AFFECTED BY AGE

Factors such as age-related decline in renal function, over-hydration or underhydration, drug-nutrient interactions, and coexisting diseases affect laboratory values.

Before age 65, serum albumin levels in men are higher than those in women, but after 65, values equalize and decline at the same rate. That rate has not been documented, but the decline in general may be due to diet.[2] The serum albumin level is, therefore, a fairly reliable measure of nutritional status in the elderly as long as hydration status and other factors are considered. In recent references, albumin levels of less than 4 g/dL in the elderly resulted in increased mortality rate.[3]

Tissue iron stores increase with age. As a result, serum transferrin levels are slightly reduced. The lower end of the normal range of serum transferrin is used in evaluating the elderly.

Blood urea nitrogen levels may rise slightly, due to the decline in renal blood flow and glomerular filtration rate.

With normal aging comes a loss of lean body mass and a decrease in creatinine excretion. To compensate for these changes, the following age-adjusted formula is used:

Men: (140 - age x kg body weight) - 72 x serum creatinine
Women (140 - age x kg body weight) - 72 x serum creatinine x 85%

Decreased hemoglobin levels are common in the elderly. It is not known whether this is due to aging per se, or to the decreased lean body mass, erythropoietin, and testosterone (in men) that occur with aging. Hemoglobin is a more direct measure of iron deficiency than hematocrit.[4] Iron deficiency follows a low iron intake, a deficient intake of vitamin C, or an excessive consumption of tea with meals. Iron absorption from the gastrointestinal (GI) tract remains intact, but transfer into the red blood cells appears defective with advancing age. This anemia is more common in elderly women than in elderly men, in those older than 75, and in housebound and nursing facility residents.

Cholesterol levels increase with age and are useful in nutrition evaluation. A cholesterol level below 160 mg/dL may indicate malnutriton.

The report by Nutrition Screening Initiative identified these major indicators of poor nutritional health in older Americans[5]:

- serum albumin less than 3.5 g/dL
- serum cholesterol less than 160 mg/dL
- serum cholesterol greater than 240 mg/dL

Aging, even without disease, changes physiology, which can alter laboratory test results. *Table 6.1* identifies laboratory tests that help registered dietitians determine the nutritional status of nursing facility residents.

Table 6.2 lists laboratory values used to describe anemias.

Table 6.1

Selected Laboratory Values*

Test	Normal values	Some implications
Albumin[5] (serum)	3.5–5.0 g/dL	*Low:* impaired hepatic synthesis (liver disease, stress, malnutrition, burns, nephrotic syndrome, overhydration, pressure ulcers, spinal cord injury, tuberculosis, cancer. Degrees of deficiency: mild = 3.2–3.5 g/dL; moderate = 2.8–3.2 g/dL; severe < 2.8 g/dL.
		Note: To interpret serum albumin levels in the elderly, use the lower end of the normal range. Serum transferrin levels do not change significantly with age.
		High: dehydration, corticosteroid therapy.
Alkaline phosphatase	20–90 IU/L	*Low:* malnutrition, scurvy, pernicious anemia, hypophosphatasia.
		High: Liver disease, bone disease.
Blood urea nitrogen (BUN)	8–20 mg/dL	With congestive heart failure, BUN may be 15–20 mg/dL.[4]
		Low: severe liver damage, low protein intake, impaired absorption, overhydration, cachexia.
		High: excessive protein intake, fever, infection, catabolism, inadequate excretion due to impaired renal function, dehydration, vomiting, diarrhea, myocardial infarction, shock, GI bleeding.
		Note: A slightly elevated BUN causes no problem unless such stresses as infection or surgery are added.[2]

* Each laboratory may use different standards to establish normal values; therefore, figures may vary among different sources.

Table 6.1 (continued)

Test	Normal values	Some implications
Calcium (serum)	8.5–10.5 mg/dL	*Low:* Severe nephritis, malabsorption syndrome (may be related to drug therapy), vitamin D deficiency, hypoparathyroidism, osteomalacia. *High:* immobilization, hyperparathyroidism, vitamin D intoxication, milk-alkali syndrome, cancer, renal calculi.
Chloride	98–109 mEq/L	*Low:* acidosis, metabolic alkalosis, vomiting, potassium deficiency, excessive sweating. *High:* anxiety states, dehydration, renal insufficiency, aspirin toxicity, nephrosis, excessive salt intake.
Cholesterol (serum)	160–250 mg/dL	*Low:* malabsorption, liver disease, hyperthyroidism, sepsis, stress, pernicious anemia, terminal stages of cancer. *Note:* Level < 160 mg/dL may be indicator of malnutriton. *High:* cardiovascular disease, obstructive jaundice, hypothyroidism, nephrosis, nephrotic syndrome.
Glucose (whole blood)	70–110 mg/dL	*Low:* pituitary hypofunction, Addison's disease, extensive liver disease, chronic renal insufficiency, alcoholism. *High:* Mild elevation: advanced age (impaired glucose tolerance 140 mg/dL fasting and 140–199 mg/dL 2 h postprandial), diuretics (thiazide and loop), cirrhosis, stress, obesity, hyperthyroidism, corticosteroids, Cushing's disease. Moderate elevation: 300–500 mg/dL, diabetes mellitus. Marked elevation: > 500 mg/dL: ketoacidosis.

Table 6.1 (continued)

Test	Normal values	Some implications
Hematocrit[5] (Hct)	M: 41%–53% F: 36%–46%	*Low:* anemia, hemorrhage, leukemia, cirrhosis, excessive fluid, hyperthyroidism. *High:* dehydration, hemoconcentration.
Hemoglobin[5] (Hgb)	M: 14–17g/dL F:12–15g/dL	*Low:* anemia (causes: deficiencies of iron, vitamins B_{12} and C, folic acid, protein; also secondary to other diseases), low serum albumin, infection, catabolism, spinal cord injury, leukemia, end-stage renal disease, poor intake of iron or intake of mainly nonheme sources, hyperthyroidism, cirrhosis, cancer, Crohn's disease, blood loss from peptic ulcer disease. *High:* hemoconcentration, dehydration following blood replacement, liver disease.
Magnesium[5] (serum)	1.3–2.0 mEq/dL	*Low:* uremia, severe diarrhea, alcoholism. *High:* chronic nephritis, liver disease. *Note:* Prolonged salicylate therapy, lithium, and magnesium-containing compounds (antacids and laxatives) falsely elevate magnesium levels, particularly if liver damage is present.
Phosphorus (serum)	2.0–4.5 mg/dL	*Low:* may occur in severe malnutrition especially during refeeding, aluminum antacid overuse. *High:* renal disease, hypoparathyroidism.

Table 6.1 (continued)

Test	Normal values	Some implications
Potassium[5] (serum)	3.5–5.0 mEq/L	*Low:* stress, surgery, uncontrolled diabetes, corticosteroids, some diuretics, vomiting, malabsorption, malnutrition, liver disease, alcohol abuse, diarrhea.
		High: renal insufficiency, intestinal obstruction, Addison's disease, catabolism, dehydration.
Prealbumin	20-50 mg/dL	*Low:* protein-energy malnutrition, metabolic stress, trauma, cirrhosis, hepatitis.
		High: patients with chronic renal failure on dialysis.
		Note: More reliable than albumin for identifying malnutrition and a more effective monitor for outcome of nutrition intervention. With adequate nutrition support it can increase by 1 mg/dL/d.[2]
Protein, total	6.0–8.4 g/dL	*Low:* Malnutrition, malabsorption, cirrhosis, steatorrhea, edema, laxative use, marasmus, leukemia.
		High: Dehydration, malignancy, Hodgkin's disease, hepatitis, leukemia, acute or chronic infections.
Prothrombin time	11–18 sec	*Prolonged:* anticoagulant therapy, liver disease, hypoprothrombinemia. No change seen in healthy elders.

Table 6.1 (continued)

Test	Normal values	Some implications
Sodium (serum)	135–145 MEq/L	*Low:* severe burns, vomiting, Addison's disease, edema, loss of bile, severe nephritis, overhydration (may cause dilutional hyponatremia), diarrhea, some diuretics, starvation, adrenal insufficiency.
		High: dehydration, inadequate fluid intake, perspiration, fever, diabetes insipidus, excessive loss of water (advanced renal disease, uncontrolled diabetes mellitus) excessive solute loading (high-protein, high-electrolyte feeding with inadequate water).
Specific gravity of urine	1.01-1.03	*High:* dehydration, diabetes, glomerulonephritis, fever, toxemia, congestive heart failure. *Note:* In the elderly specific gravity may decline because of a 33%-50% decline in the number of nephrons, which can impair the kidney's ability to concentrate urine.
Total lymphocyte count (TLC)	3000–3500 cells/mm^3	*Low:* corticosteroid therapy, cancer, chemotherapy, radiotherapy, surgery, lymphopenia, malnutrition.
		Degrees of depletion: mild = 1500–1800; moderate = 900–1500; Severe <900.
		High: leukemia, infectious bacterial diseases, leukocytosis.

Table 6.1 (continued)

Test	Normal values	Some implications
Transferrin[5] (serum)	180–380 g/dL	*Low:* malnutrition, cirrhosis, hepatitis nephrotic syndrome, overhydration, pernicious anemia, chronic infection.
		High: iron deficiency anemia, dehydration.
		Note: Transferrin saturation (percentage) is useful in detecting decreased iron stores. Deficiency levels < 20% in men; < 15% in women.
Triglycerides (serum)	40–150 mg/dL	*Low:* malnutrition, congenital hypolipoproteinemia.
		High: liver disease, nephrotic syndrome, hypothyroidism, poorly controlled diabetes, pancreatitis, glycogen storage disease, myocardial infarction, hyperlipoproteinemias, alcohol abuse.

Table 6.2

Laboratory Values Used in Describing Anemias

Test	Microcytic hypochromic*	Macrocytic†	Anemia or chronic disease
Red blood cells (RBC)	Normal (4.0–5.5 million)	Low	Low
Hgb	Low	Low	Low
Hct	Low	Low	Low
Mean corpuscular volume (MCV)	Low <80 μm^3	High > 94 μm^3	Normal 80–94 μm^3
Mean corpuscular hemoglobin (MCH)	Low < 27 pg	High > 32 pg	Normal 27–32 pg
Mean corpuscular hemoglobin concentration (MCHC)	Low < 30%	Normal >30%	Normal >30%
Total iron binding capacity (TIBC) Normal = 250–400 mg/dL	High	Low	Low

* Iron deficiency
† B$_{12}$, folate deficiency.

Hemoglobin is the oxygen-carrying, iron-containing protein in the blood. Hematocrit measures the percentage of packed red cells in a volume of whole blood. The blood smear is then examined to determine the size and color of the red blood cells. The cells are then counted and grouped by size and the amount of hemoglobin present. From this the following three values are derived. Mean cell volume (MCV) estimates the average size of the red blood cell. Mean cell hemoglobin (MCH) measures the average amount of hemoglobin per cell. Mean cell hemoglobin concentration (MCHC) is the ratio of hemoglobin and hematocrit readings.

In the microcytic anemia of iron deficiency, all three derived values are low. In the macrocytic anemia due to a deficiency of folic acid or vitamin B_{12}, the MCV is high or normal, and the MCH and MCHC may be normal or high. This means the cells are larger than normal and laden with hemoglobin.

References

1. Abrahams WB, Berkaw R, Fletcher AJ. *The Merck Manual of Geriatrics*. Rahway, NJ: Merck Sharp and Dohme Research Laboratories; 1990:1167–1188.
2. *Pocket Resource for Nutrition Assessment*. Chicago, Ill: Consultant Dietitians in Health Care Facilities: Dietetic Practice Group; 1990.
3. Rudman D, Peller AG. Protein-calorie undernutrition in the nursing home. *J Am Geriatr Soc*. 1989;37:173–183.
4. Grant A, DeHoog S. *Nutritional Assessment and Support*. 4th ed. Seattle, Wash: Grant and DeHoog; 1991:99–152.
5. *Report of Nutrition Screening 1: Toward a Common View*. Washington, DC: Nutrition Screening Initiative; 1991.
6. *Interpretive Guidelines for Long Term Care Facilities*. Washington, DC: Health Care Financing Administration; 1992.

Food-Medication Interactions

Medications can be affected by foods ingested, and medications can affect nutritional status. The question of drugs and nutrition, and their interrelationship becomes pertinent, since nutrition plays a vital role in the medical services available for residents. Vulnerability to drug-induced nutritional deficiencies is greatest in the elderly, the chronically ill and anyone with marginal or inadequate nutrient intake. At special risk are those residents who are under long-term drug therapy or stress. Without proper nutrition management, elderly residents may be subject to nutrient depletion or altered drug response.

The following classifications of commonly prescribed drugs and over-the-counter drugs are most often used by these vulnerable groups. The related food-medication interactions are described along with their nutrition implications, possible side effects, and dietary cautions. *Note:* Each drug should be checked for its unique interactions and altered laboratory values.

Drug Classification: Antiarrhythmics and Vasodilators

Examples: verapamil (Calan), diltiazem (Cardizem), encainide (Enkaid), procainamide (Pronestyl), and amrinone lactate (Inocor), hydralazine (Apresoline)

Administration	Dietary suggestions	Nutrition implications	Gastrointestinal symptoms	Special conditions	Metabolic/ physiologic	Other effects	Supplements
Oral or parenteral. Take 1 hour before or 2 hours after a meal.	Caution with herbal teas. Avoid natural licorice. Diet high in potassium, low in sodium and adequate in magnesium and calcium recommended.	Monitor electrolytes, especially potassium. May contain lactose; check each drug.	Constipation, anorexia, nausea.	Avoid alcohol. Caution with diabetes: glucose absorption is inhibited. Do dental care cautiously.	Edema.	Vomiting, dizziness, heartburn, blurred vision, abnormal taste and smell, diarrhea, dyspepsia, headache, dry mouth, fatigue, tremor.	Avoid those with vitamin D or calcium, as they reduce drug effects.

Drug Classification: Anticoagulants

Examples: warfarin sodium (Coumadin), heparin sodium (Heparin)

Administration	Dietary suggestions	Nutrition implications	Gastrointestinal symptoms	Special conditions	Metabolic/ physiologic	Other effects	Supplements
Oral or parenteral.	Need for balanced diet with consistent vitamin K intake: an increase reduces drug effectiveness; a decrease increases anticoagulant effect. Avoid proteolytic enzymes (papain), soybean oil, fried or boiled onions, all of which increase fibrinolytic activity. Limit green and herbal teas. Limit caffeine.	Cooking oils with silicone additive decrease drug absorption.	Diarrhea, GI pain and cramps, constipation.	Avoid alcohol. Do dental care cautiously. Hyperkalemia.	Blood dyscrasias. Hepatitis or jaundice.	Bloating; anorexia; headache; dizziness; black; tarry stools.	Vitamins A, E, K, and C may alter prothrombin time.

Drug Classification: Anticonvulsant Agents

Examples: phenytoin sodium (Dilantin), valproic acid (Depakene), primidone (Mysoline), phenobarbital

Administration	Dietary suggestions	Nutrition implications	Gastrointestinal symptoms	Special conditions	Metabolic/ physiologic	Other effects	Supplements
Take with food to lower GI distress.	Caution with calcium, pyridoxine, folacin.	*Phenytoin*—low bioavailability of drug with tube feeding. *Primidone*—low calcium absorption. *Phenobarbital*—low serum levels vitamins B$_{12}$ and C, folacin, phyidoxine, calcium, magnesium.	Nausea, vomiting, diarrhea, epigastric pain, constipation.	Avoid alcohol. Caution with diabetes. Do dental care cautiously.	Blood dyscrasias, pancreatitis, edema, decreased bone density.	Dizziness, headache, confusion, decreased appetite and weight, visual changes, altered taste, drowsiness, anorexia.	*Phenytoin*:—calcium may lower bioavailability of both drug and mineral.

Drug Classification: βAdrenergic Blocking Agents

Examples: propranolol (Inderal), timolol maleate (Blocadren), pindolol (Visken), acebutolol (Sectral), penbutolol sulfate (Levatol), metoprolol tartrate (Lopressor), esmolol (Brevibloc), betaxolol (Kerlone), atenolol (Tenormin)

Administration	Dietary suggestions	Nutrition implications	Gastrointestinal symptoms	Special conditions	Metabolic/ physiologic	Other effects	Supplements
Take with food to increase drug availability.	Low-sodium, low-calorie diet for hypertension. Limit natural licorice. Avoid caffeine.	May contain lactose; check each drug.	Constipation or diarrhea, nausea, vomiting.	Limit alcohol. Monitor diabetic residents: hypoglycemia can persist.	Edema.	Anorexia, bitter taste, dizziness, dry mouth, fatigue, sore throat, heartburn and gastric distress.	Take no iron or magnesium within 2 hours of taking drug.

Drug Classification: Cardiovascular Drugs

Examples: (cardiotonic) digoxin (Digoxin, Lanoxin), digitoxin (Crystodigin)

Administration	Dietary suggestions	Nutrition implications	Gastrointestinal symptoms	Special conditions	Metabolic/ physiologic	Other effects	Supplements
Oral or parenteral. Take with water 1 hour before or 2 hours after high-fiber foods.	Maintain diet high in potassium, low in sodium, and adequate in calcium and magnesium. Avoid natural licorice.	Glucose absorption may be inhibited. Elixir is incompatible with enteral formulas. Tablets may contain lactose.	Nausea, vomiting, diarrhea.	Caution with herbal teas.	Monitor electrolytes for imbalance.	Anorexia, decreased weight, blurred vision, drowsiness, headache, weakness. Note: 25% of persons older than 70 and taking digoxin lose weight.	Calcium- and vitamin D-induced hypercalcemia may potentiate drug effects and result in cardiac arrhythmias.

Drug Classification: Cardiovascular Drugs

Examples: (diuretics) furosemide (Lasix), methyclothiazide (Aquatensen, Enduron), acetazolamide (Diamox), bumetanide (Bumex), ethacrynic acid (Edecrin), Mannitol, metolazone (Diulo, Zaroxolyn), quinethazone (Hydromox), triamterene (Dyrenium), spironolactone (Aldactone)

Administration	Dietary suggestions	Nutrition implications	Gastrointestinal symptoms	Special conditions	Metabolic/ physiologic	Other effects	Supplements
Oral or parenteral. Food reduces absorption: take on empty stomach. May take food to reduce GI distress.	Low-calorie, low-sodium, high-potassium diet. Do not mix with acidic solutions. Avoid natural licorice, salt substitutes.	Triamterene reduces utilization of dietary folacin and conserves potassium. May contain lactose.	Nausea, vomiting, cramps.	Avoid alcohol. Monitor diabetic residents: reduces carbohydrate tolerance.	Blood dyscrasias. Pancreatitis. Electrolyte imbalance with reduced potassium.	Dizziness, anorexia, dry mouth, peculiar sweet taste, headache, thirst, drowsiness, blurred vision.	

Drug Classification: Antihyperlipemic Agents (cholesterol-lowering drugs)

Examples: cholestyramine (Questran), colestipol (Colestid), nicotinic acid (Nicobid), gemfibrozil (Lopid), lavastatin (Mevacor), probucol (Lorelco)

Administration	Dietary suggestions	Nutrition implications	Gastrointestinal symptoms	Special conditions	Metabolic/ physiologic	Other effects	Supplements
Take with moist foods or water (never dry). Do not take with carbonated beverages.	Fat-modified, low-cholesterol, increased fluid and fiber diet. Follow prescribed diet. With dextrothyroxine avoid large amounts of goiterogenic foods.	Reduced absorption of calcium, fat; vitamins A, D, and B₁₂; folacin; medium chain triglycerides; and glucose. Iron reserves reduced in long-term use.	Constipation.	Monitor diabetic residents: carbohydrate tolerance is reduced.	Monitor triglycerides and cholesterol. Edema, osteomalacia, jaundice, or anemia.	Flatulence, heartburn, nausea, GI bleeding and pain, dizziness, blurred vision, belching, diarrhea, steatorrhea, anorexia, increased or decreased weight, altered taste acuity, drowsiness.	Do not use vitamin supplements as substitute for balanced diet.

Drug Classification: Gastrointestinal Medications

Examples: (Antisecretory or antiulcer) cimetidine (Tagamet), dicyclomine (Bentyl), nizatidine (Axid), famotidine (Pepcid), (Librax), misoprostol (Cytotec), omeprazole (Prilosec), ranitidine (Zantac)

Administration	Dietary suggestions	Nutrition implications	Gastrointestinal symptoms	Special conditions	Metabolic/physiologic	Other effects	Supplements
Oral or parenteral. Take with food.	Avoid any irritating foods, beverages, seasonings.	Reduced folacin and vitamin B$_{12}$ absorption. Iron salts reduce drug absorption and gastric secretion.	Constipation	Limit xanthine-containing foods. Limit alcohol. Do dental care cautiously.	Monitor for hyperglycemia.	Headache, dry mouth, drowsiness, altered taste, heartburn, blurred vision, abdominal pain, diarrhea, nausea, vomiting, dizziness, confusion (especially in elderly), fatigue, increased weight.	

Drug Classification: Gastrointestinal Medications

Examples: (laxatives) bisacodyl (Dulcolax), phenolphthalein (Ex-Lax), mineral oil, psyllium (Fiberall, Metamucil, Perdiem)

Administration	Dietary suggestions	Nutrition implications	Gastrointestinal symptoms	Special conditions	Metabolic/physiologic	Other effects	Supplements
Take on empty stomach with water. Increase fluid intake. Swallow whole. Do not take within 1 hour of dairy products.	Increase fiber in diet.	Reduced intestinal absorption of glucose. *Mineral oil*—reduced absorption of vitamins A, D, E, and K; carotene; calcium; and phosphorus.	None.	Caution with diabetes.	Hypokalemia.	Abdominal cramps, belching, diarrhea, nausea. *Mineral oil*—decreased weight, anorexia, chalky taste, flatulence.	

Drug Classification: Central Nervous System Medications and Psychotherapeutics

Examples: (tricyclic antidepressants) amitriptyline (Elavil, Endep), amoxapine (Asendin), desipramine (Norpramin), doxepin (Sinequan), clomipramine (Anafranil), nortriptyline (Pamelor), protriptyline

Administration	Dietary suggestions	Nutrition implications	Gastrointestinal symptoms	Special conditions	Metabolic/physiologic	Other effects	Supplements
Oral or parenteral. Take with food to reduce GI distress.	Increased appetite for sweets.	Increased need for riboflavin.	Constipation, nausea, dry mouth, blurred vision, dizziness.	Avoid alcohol. Limit caffeine. Do dental care with caution.	Syndrome of inappropriate secretion of antidiuretic hormone. Blood dyscrasia. Edema.	Nausea, vomiting, altered taste, increased or decreased weight, lactation, drowsiness, headache, confusion (especially in elderly).	

Drug Classification: Central Nervous System Medications and Psychotherapeutics

Examples: (lithium) lithium carbonate (Eskalith, Lithane, Lithobid)

Administration	Dietary suggestions	Nutrition implications	Gastrointestinal symptoms	Special conditions	Metabolic/physiologic	Other effects	Supplements
Take with food. Drink 2 to 3 qt water or fluids daily.	Avoid dietary extremes. A constant sodium intake is the key to stable lithium levels. Know sodium content of foods eaten.	None.	None	Limit caffeine. Caution with diabetes.	Reduced calcium uptake by bone. Monitor electrolytes. Edema.	Nausea, vomiting, diarrhea, bloating, metallic or altered taste, increased weight, increased thirst, dry mouth, blurred vision, dizziness, drowsiness.	

Drug Classification: Central Nervous System Medications and Psychotherapeutics

Examples: (monoamine oxidase inhibitor) isocarboxazid (Marplan), phenelzine (Nardil), tranylcypromine (Parnate)

Administration	Dietary suggestions	Nutrition implications	Gastrointestinal symptoms	Special conditions	Metabolic/physiologic	Other effects	Supplements
None.	Avoid foods high in pressor amines (eg, aged cheese, wine, yogurt, meat extracts). Limit caffeine.	May contain lactose; check each drug.	Constipation, dizziness.	Avoid alcohol. Monitor diabetic residents: increased hypoglycemic effect.	Edema, fluid and electrolyte imbalance. Jaundice. Blood dyscrasias. Syndrome of inappropriate secretion of antidiuretic hormone.	Gastrointestinal distress and pain, drowsiness, anorexia, decreased or increased weight, nausea, tremors, dry mouth, blurred vision, headache.	Tryptophan may result in headache, hypertension.

Drug Classification: Central Nervous System Medications and Psychotherapeutics

Examples: (Antiparkinsonism) carbidopa-levodopa (Sinemet), amantadine (Symmetrel), benztropine (Cogentin), bromocriptine (Parlodel) levodopa (Larodopa), trihexyphenidyl (Artane), pergolide (Permax), selegiline (Eldepryl)

Administration	Dietary suggestions	Nutrition implications	Gastrointestinal symptoms	Special conditions	Metabolic/physiologic	Other effects	Supplements
Oral or parenteral. Take with food to reduce GI upset.	*Limit pyridoxine to 10 mg per day. Increased need of vitamins C and B₁₂. Do not take with hydrolysates. Levodopa*—do not take with high-protein food. Distribute protein equally throughout day and do not ingest with drug. *Selegiline*—avoid food high in tyramine.	None.	Nausea, dizziness, epigastric distress.	Avoid alcohol. Do dental care cautiously. Avoid caffeine. *Levodopa*—monitor diabetic residents: blood glucose may be altered.	Edema.	Fatigue, vomiting, constipation or diarrhea, confusion, dry mouth, hiccups, abdominal cramps, headache, drowsiness, blurred vision, anorexia.	5 mg pyridoxine per day may reduce levodopa effects.

Drug Classification: Respiratory Tract Agents, Bronchodilators

Examples: albuterol sulfate (Proventil, Ventolin), metaproterenol (Alupent, Metaprel), aminophylline (Aminophylline), (Asbron), theophylline (Bronkodyl, SloBid, Theobid), oxtriphylline (Choledyl), dyphylline (Dilor, Lufyllin), terbutaline sulfate (Brethine, Bricanyl), ipratropium bromide (Atrovent), ephedrine (Marax), (Tedral)

Administration	Dietary suggestions	Nutrition implications	Gastrointestinal symptoms	Special conditions	Metabolic/physiologic	Other effects	Supplements
Oral or parenteral. Take with water 1 hour before or 2 hours after meals.	*Theophylline*—avoid charcoal-broiled foods. Avoid extremes of dietary protein and carbohydrates. *Dyphylline*—limit caffeine. Not affected by charcoal-broiled foods.	May contain lactose; check each drug. Elixir containing sorbitol may cause diarrhea.	Tremors.	Do dental care cautiously. *Marax*: avoid alcohol.	Syndrome of inappropriate antidiuretic hormone. Caution with diabetes; possible hyperglycemia. Hypermetabolism.	Nausea, vomiting, epigastric pain, diarrhea, drowsiness, dizziness, anorexia, bitter aftertaste, headache.	

Calan is manufactured by G.D. Searle and Co, Chicago, IL 60680; Cardizem, Marion Merrell Dow, Kansas City, MO 64114; Enkaid, Bristol Laboratories, Evansville, IN 47721; Inocor, Sanofi Winthrop Pharmaceuticals, New York, NY 10016; Pronestyl, Princeton, NJ 08543; Apresoline, Ciba Pharmaceuticals, Summit, NJ 07901.

Coumadin, DuPont Pharmaceuticals, Wilmington, DE 19880; Heparin, Elkins-Sinn Inc, Cherry Hill, NJ 08003.

Dilantin, Parke-Davis, Morris Plains, NJ 07950; Depakene, Abbott Laboratories, North Chicago, IL 60064; Mysoline, Wyeth-Ayerst, Philadelphia, PA 19101.

Inderal, Wyeth-Ayerst; Blocadren, Merck Sharp and Dohme, West Point, PA 19486; Visken, Sandoz Pharmaceuticals, East Hanover, NJ 07936; Sectral, Wyeth-Ayerst; Levatol, Reed and Carnrick, Jersey City, NJ 07302; Lopressor, Geigy, Ardsley, NY 10502; Brevibloc, DuPont Pharmaceuticals; Kerlone, G. D. Searle and Co; Tenormin, ICI Pharma, Wilmington, DE 19897.

Digoxin, Roxane, Columbus, OH 43228; Lanoxin, Burroughs Wellcome, Research Triangle Park, NC 27709; Crystodigin, Eli Lilly and Co, Indianapolis, IN 46285.

Lasix, Hoechst-Roussel, Somerville, NJ 00876; Aquatensen, Wallace, Cranbury, NJ 08512; Enduron, Abbott Laboratories; Diamox, Lederle, Wayne, NJ 07470; Bumex, Roche Laboratories, Nutley, NJ 07110; Edecrin, Merck Sharp and Dohme; Diulo, Schiapparelli Searle, Chicago, IL 60680; Zaroxolyn, Fisons Pharmaceuticals, Rochester, NY 14623; Hydromox, Lederle; Dyrenium, SmithKline Beecham Pharmaceuticals, Philadelphia, PA 19101; Aldactone, G. D. Searle and Co.

Questran, Bristol Laboratories; Colestid, Upjohn, Kalamazoo, MI 49001; Nicobid, Rhone-Poulenc Rorer Pharmaceuticals, Collegeville, PA 19426; Lopid, Parke-Davis; Mevacor, Merck Sharp and Dohme; Lorelco, Marion Merrell Dow.

Tagamet, SmithKline Beecham; Bentyl, Marion Merrell Dow; Axid, Eli Lilly and Co; Pepcid, Merck Sharp and Dohme; Librax, Roche Products, Manati, PR 00674; Cytotec, G. D. Searle and Co; Prilosec, Merck Sharp and Dohme; Zantac, Glaxo Pharmaceuticals, Research Triangle Park, NC 27709.

Dulcolax, Ciba Consumer, Edison, NJ 08837; Ex-Lax, Sandoz Consumer, East Hanover, NJ 07936; Fiberall, Ciba Consumer; Metamucil, Procter and Gamble, Cincinnati, OH 45201; Perdiem, Rhone-Poulenc Rorer Consumer.

Elavil, Stuart Pharmaceuticals, Wilmington, DE 19897; Endep, Roche Products; Asendin, Lederle; Norpramin, Marion Merrell Dow; Sinequan, Roerig, New York, NY 10017; Anafranil, Basel, Sumit, NJ 07901; Pamelor, Sandoz Pharmaceuticals.

Eskalith, SmithKline Beecham; Lithane, Miles Pharmaceuticals, West Haven, CT 06516; Lithobid, Ciba Pharmaceuticals.

Marplan, Roche Laboratories; Nardil, Parke-Davis; Parnate, SmithKline Beecham.

Sinemet, DuPont Pharmaceuticals; Symmetrel, DuPont Multi-Source Products, Garden City, NY 11530; Cogentin, Merck Sharp and Dohme; Parlodel, Sandoz Pharmaceuticals; Larodopa, Roche Laboratories; Artane, Lederle; Permax, Eli Lilly and Co; Eldepryl, Denville, NJ 07834.

Proventil, Schering, Kenilworth, NJ 07033; Ventolin, Allen and Hanburys, Research Triangle Park, NC 27709; Alupent, Boehringer Ingelheim, Ridgefield, CT 06877; Metaprel, Sandoz Pharmaceuticals; Aminophyllin, G. D. Searle; Asbron, Sandoz Pharmaceuticals; BronKodyl, Sanofi Winthrop Pharmaceuticals; Slo-bid, Rhone-Poulenc Rorer; Choledyl, Parke-Davis; Dilor, Savage, Melville, NY 11747; Lufyllin, Wallace; Brethine, Geigy; Bricanyl, Marion Merrell Dow; Atrovent, Boehringer Ingelheim; Marax, Roerig; Tedral, Parke-Davis.

Alcohol

Chronic alcohol intake stimulates the microsomal system responsible for the metabolism of many drugs and may cause a variety of adverse effects. Ethanol is absorbed from the alimentary canal, metabolized by the liver, and may be distributed throughout the body tissues and fluids. Absorption can be affected by the type of beverage consumed, pH of the GI tract, alcohol concentration, and concomitant ingestion of food. Individual variation in pharmacokinetics of alcohol result from differences in hepatic function, renal function, body mass, fat, and water content. Depending on the quantity of alcohol consumed and the time of ingestion, the biotransformation of some drugs can be increased or decreased. Some unusual effects of taking certain drugs and alcohol at the same time include unpredictable fluctuations of plasma glucose concentrations and a disulfiram-like reaction in residents who use oral hypoglycemic agents. In the latter case, the drug alters the intermediary metabolism of alcohol, thus causing an accumulation of acetaldehyde. The signs and symptoms of disulfiram-like reaction are flushing, pulsating headache, respiratory difficulties, nausea, vomiting, and hypotension. Residents should be warned to watch for hidden sources of alcohol such as flavoring agents and extracts added to food after cooking, uncooked fermented foods and sauces, and over-the-counter medications containing alcohol.

Nutrient-Drug Interactions

Table 6.3 shows drug interactions with vitamins, minerals, and other food supplements. The potential exists for adverse drug effect in medicated residents who use food supplements concurrently and indiscriminately.

Table 6.3

Food Supplements and Drug Interactions

Supplements	Drug	Effect
Vitamins		
A	Aluminum hydroxide	Drug-induced precipitated bile acids may decrease vitamin absorption.
	Cholestyramine	Concurrent use may impair vitamin absorption.
	Mineral oil	Concurrent use may interfere with vitamin absorption.
	Warfarin	Large doses may enhance anticoagulant activity.
D	Digoxin	Vitamin D-induced hypercalcemia may sensitize resident to toxic effects of drug.
	Mineral oil, aluminum hydroxide, cholestyramine	Concurrent use may decrease vitamin absorption.
E	Warfarin	Megadoses may enhance anticoagulant activity.
	Mineral oil, aluminum hydroxide, cholestyramine	Concurrent use may decrease vitamin absorption.
K	Warfarin	Concurrent use inhibits hypoprothrombic effect of drug.
	Mineral oil, aluminum hydroxide, cholestyramine	Concurrent use may decrease vitamin absorption.
Ascorbic acid	Haloperidol	Concurrent use may enhance antipsychotic effect of drug.
	Warfarin	Megadoses may decrease prothrombin time.
B_{12} (cobalamin)	Cimetidine Neomycin	Concurrent use may reduce absorption of vitamin.
Folacin	Phenytoin	Vitamin replacement in folate-deficient residents may increase drug metabolism.
Pyridoxine	Levodopa	Concurrent use reverses antiparkinsonian effect.
	Phenytoin	Large doses may reduce anticonvulsant activity.
	Hydralazine, isoniazid, penicillamine	Concurrent use may reverse drug-induced peripheral neuropathy.
Thiamin	Aluminum hydroxide	Inactivated by drug.
Minerals		
Calcium	Digitalis	Concurrent use with vitamin D may result in hypercalcemia and may enhance toxic effects of drug.
	Hydrochlorothiazide	Concurrent use with vitamin D may result in hypercalcemia.
	Laxatives (abuse)	Reduced absorption.
	Phenytoin	Concurrent use may decrease both drug and calcium bioavailability.

Table 6.3 (continued)

Food Supplements and Drug Interactions

Supplements	Drug	Effect
Minerals	Verapamil	Concurrent use with vitamin D may counter the antidysrhythmic effect of drug.
Copper	Penicillamine	May induce mineral depletion.
Iron	Penicillamine	Concurrent use may decrease drug effectiveness.
	Non-narcotic analgesics (aspirin, indomethacin)	May aggrevate or contribute to iron deficiency anemia (4–5 g daily in long-term use causes 3–8 mL fecal blood loss).
	Calcium carbonate	Concurrent use may impair iron absorption.
Magnesium	Ethanol	Reduced absorption.
Phosphorus	Antacids	Reduced absorption.
Potassium	Furosemide, hydrochlorothiazide, spironolactone	Monitor for abnormal levels.
	Ethanol	Reduced absorption.
	Diuretics	Reduced absorption.
	Laxatives (abuse)	Reduced absorption.
Zinc	Penicillamine	Reduced absorption.
	Ethanol	Reduced absorption.
Other Supplements		
Protein or amino acids	Levodopa, methyldopa	Concurrent use may potentially inhibit drug absorption.
	Theophylline	Concurrent use may potentially decrease plasma half-life of drug.
Tryptophan	Fluoxetine	Concurrent use may intensify agitation, restlessness, and GI problems.
	Monoamine oxidase inhibitors (MAOI)	Concurrent use may result in confusion, deterioration in mental status, headaches, agitation, and other adverse effects.
	Tricyclic antidepressants	Variable results are observed when used to augment antidepressant effects.

Adapted from Smith CH. Drug-food/food-drug interactions. In: *Geriatric Nutrition*. New York, NY: The Raven Press Ltd; 1990;29:392.

Summary

The benefits of recognizing food-medication interactions are as follows:

- Increased drug effectiveness reduces cost of health care service.
- Reduced charges to the resident by reducing hospital days.
- Decreased labor and food costs from reduction in modified diets and expensive nourishments.
- Improved meal consumption by residents, resulting in less plate waste.
- Less liability by recognizing possible adverse reactions.
- Identification of malnutrition which is classified as a co-morbidity under the diagnosis related groups (DRGs).

The impact of drugs on nutritional status and the effects of food, modified diets, and dietary habits on drug action have to be evaluated on an individual basis. The registered dietitian and pharmacist are uniquely qualified to do this evaluation. The registered dietitian has the skills to identify the malnourished resident and intercede with improved nutrition care, which can be cost effective to the facility.

Recommendations Concerning Supplement Usage: ADA Statement

In 1987 The American Dietetic Association was responsible for attaining agreement on a statement for vitamin and mineral supplement usage from the American Institute of Nutrition, the American Society for Clinical Nutrition, and the National Council Against Health Fraud. The American Medical Association's Council on Scientific Affairs reviewed the statement and found it to be consistent with its official statement on dietary supplements.

The Task Force statement regarding vitamin and mineral supplement usage is[14]:

Healthy children and adults should obtain adequate nutrient intakes from dietary sources. Meeting nutrient needs by choosing a variety of foods in moderation, rather than by supplementation, reduces the potential risk for both nutrient deficiencies and nutrient excesses. Individual recommendations regarding supplements and diets should come from physicians and registered dietitians.

Supplement usage may be indicated in some circumstances including:

Women with excessive menstrual bleeding may need to take iron supplements.

Women who are pregnant or breastfeeding need more of certain nutrients, especially iron, folic acid, and calcium.

People with very low calorie intakes frequently consume diets that do not meet their needs for all nutrients.

Some vegetarians may not be receiving adequate calcium, iron, zinc, and vitamin B_{12}.

Newborns are commonly given, under the direction of a physician, a single dose of vitamin K to prevent abnormal bleeding.

Certain disorders or diseases and some medications may interfere with nutrient intake, digestion, absorption, metabolism, or excretion and thus change requirements.

Nutrients are potentially toxic when ingested in sufficiently large amounts. Safe intake levels vary widely from nutrient to nutrient and may vary with the age and health of the individual. In addition, high dosage vitamin and mineral supplements can interfere with the normal metabolism of other nutrients and with the therapeutic effects of certain drugs.

The Recommended Dietary Allowances represent the best currently available assessment of safe and adequate intakes, and serve as the basis for the US Recommended Daily Allowances shown on many product labels. There are no demonstrated benefits of self-supplementation beyond these allowances.

In the elderly population, taking vitamin and mineral supplements unnecessarily is commonplace. As Hess states, "the increasing belief that high-dose single-nutrient supplements will promote good health or prevent disease suggests some Americans may be setting themselves up for potential vitamin or mineral overdose."[14]

Vitamins A, B_6, C, and D and the minerals zinc and selenium carry the highest potential for toxicity and severity of overdose symptoms. Hess further states, "these supplements, consumed frequently and in large doses, in addition to foods provide an intake many times the Recommended Dietary Allowances and may risk health problems. Food is the best and safest source of nutrients. It is far better to improve your diet than to rely on supplements to promote health."[14]

Therefore, in the nursing facility the registered dietitian promotes optimal nutritional status for the resident through the intake of food to improve the quality of life.

References

1. Allen AM. *Food-Medication Interactions.* 7th ed. Tempe, Az: AM Allen; 1991.
2. Cerrato PL. Drugs and food: when the dangers increase. *RN.* Nov 1988:65–67.
3. Clinical Report On Aging. *J Am Geriatr Soc.* 1988;2:18.
4. Powers DE, Moore AO. The costs of food medication interactions. *The Consultant Dietitian.* 1986;11:4:9–12.
5. Holt V, Nordstrom J, Kohrs MB. Food preferences of older adults. *J Nutr Elderly.* 1989; 6:3:47–55.
6. Lamy PP. Effects of diet and nutrition on drug therapy. *J Am Geriatr Soc.* 1982;30:11:30–99.
7. Lamy PO. A consideration of NSAID use in the elderly. *Geriatric Med Today.* 1988;7:4.
8. Morley JE. Institutionalized death by starvation. Presented at 74th Annual Meeting of The American Dietetic Association. Dallas, Tex; Oct. 1991.
9. Nutrition and drug therapy for the elderly. *Nutrition Food Aging.* 1987;7:1–3.
10. Randle NW. Food or nutrient effects on drug absorption: a review. *Hosp Pharm.* 1987;22:694–697.
11. Roe DA. Therapeutic effects of drug-nutrient interactions in the elderly. *J Am Diet Assoc.* 1985;85:174.
12. Roe DA. Dimensions of risk assessment for drug and nutrient interactions. *Nutr Today.* Nov/Dec 1987: 20–25.
13. Smith CH. Dietary concerns associated with the use of medications. *J Am Diet Assoc.* 1984;84:901.

14. Recommendations concerning supplement usage: ADA statement. *J Am Diet Assoc.* 1987;87:1342–1343.
15. Smith CH. Drug-food/food-drug interactions. In: *Geriatric Nutrition.* New York, NY: Raven Press, Ltd; 1990; 29:392.
16. Stein EM, Stein S, Linn MW. Geriatric sweet tooth. *J Am Geriatr Soc.* 1985;33:687.
17. Roe DA. *Geriatric Nutrition.* 3rd ed. Englewood Cliffs, NJ: Prentice Hall; 1990:199.

Enteral and Parenteral Feedings

Residents in nursing facilities often require nutrition support to supply adequate calories, protein, and other nutrients when they are unable or unwilling to eat.[1] Nutrition support can be defined as the provision of nutrients via specialized formulas and solutions to meet the requirements of nutritionally compromised residents.

It has been estimated that 2% of the elderly population in nursing facilities require either enteral or parenteral support. The number of malnourished elderly residents requiring nutrition support is expected to increase as the elderly population is predicted to double by the year 2040.[2,3] When warranted, the registered dietitian can help residents derive maximum benefit from medical therapy by making nutrition support an integral component of that therapy. This section is designed to describe the different types of nutrition support available and their application.

Enteral Nutrition Support

Enteral nutrition can be divided into two categories, an oral diet and oral supplements, or tube feedings.

ORAL DIET

Many residents can meet their nutritional requirements with the standard house diet. Those residents with mildly increased protein or caloric needs may be met with fortification of menu items to reach a desired level of nutrient density such as addition of evaporated milk, cream, margarine, gravies, and sauces to appropriate foods. Others may benefit from a type of oral supplement between meals. In selecting an oral supplement, factors to consider are nutrient density, flavor, texture, and special nutrient needs. Usually the resident is in need of additional calories and protein due to significant weight loss or pressure ulcers. Increased intake may be accomplished by offering the resident nutrient-dense food choices between meals, such as a half sandwich, milk, fortified milk, milk toast, custard, pudding, ice cream, or some other favorite food. A variety of nutritional supplements available in the health care market can meet these increased needs.[3] Taste is important for good acceptability and optimal intake. To optimize these factors it is recommended the flavors be varied to avoid flavor fatigue; the texture be altered, and in some cases bland or less sweet formulations be used because of the aversion to sweet tastes. Specialized oral supplements have been formulated to meet special nutrient requirements. Examples of these are: nutritionally complete puddings, which dysphagic residents may find easier to swallow than liquids; calorically dense, low-protein supplements for residents with renal dysfunction; and lactose-free products for residents with lactose intolerance. There also may be a need for a modular supplement, which provides a single nutrient. For example, a carbohydrate supplement is used for residents who require increased calories only and no other nutrients; or protein supplementation may be indicated when metabolic stress causes a significant protein loss.[4]

TUBE FEEDING

Often residents cannot meet their nutrition requirements with an oral diet secondary to increased metabolic demands or decreased appetite or ability to eat. In these residents, enteral tube feedings can either supplement or provide total nutrition support. Upon admission to a nursing facility, a malnourished resident may greatly benefit from a temporary tube feeding. *Table 6.4* lists additional indications for tube feeding.

Table 6.4

Indications for Tube Feedings

Enteral
- Admitting diagnosis of malnutrition or undernutrition
- Five to seven days of oral intake of 50% or less
- Severe protein-energy malnutrition (neoplasm, inflammation, trauma, burns, chemotherapy, radiation)
- Coma or depressed mental status
- Unintentional weight loss of more than 10% of usual body weight in 6 months
- Unplanned weight loss of 5% in 1 month or less
- Severe pressure sores (stage III or IV)
- Neurologic or psychiatric disorders (often resulting in dysphagia)
- Chronic aspiration
- Abnormality of GI tract (pancreatitis, fistula, short bowel syndrome, malabsorption, inflammatory bowel disease)

Total Parenteral Nutrition
- Abnormality of GI tract (massive small bowel resection)
- Ingestion of food is impossible (obstruction)
- Intractable diarrhea or vomiting
- Impaired digestion and absorption; eg, malabsorption, radiation enteritis, or ulcerative colitis
- Trauma to the gut; eg, short bowel syndrome, edema due to severe malnutrition
- Receiving high-dose chemotherapy, radiation, and/or bone marrow transplantation

Tube feedings can be provided with a nutritionally complete formula delivered into a functioning GI tract via a tube.[5] If a resident cannot digest or absorb the formula, another method of nutrition support is warranted.

Residents who require tube feeding receive formula through a nasogastric, nasoduodenal, nasojejunal, esophagostomy, gastrostomy, or jejunostomy tube.[6,7] A nasogastric tube should be used for short term. It is recommended for long-term feeding that the permanent tube be an esophagostomy, gastrostomy, or jejunostomy.

FORMULAS

A wide range of formulas now exists. Formulas differ in composition but generally are nutritionally complete when supplied in amounts sufficient to meet caloric needs. There are three basic types of enteral formulas: polymeric, predigested, and modular.

Polymeric formulas are the most common and frequently used formulas. They contain intact forms of protein, carbohydrates, and fat. This necessitates normal GI tract functioning.

The *predigested formulas* (chemically defined or elemental) have one or more nutrients that have been partially digested. This helps ease digestion and absorption in residents with compromised GI tracts.

In *modular formulas* individual nutrients (ie, protein, fat, carbohydrates, vitamins, and minerals) are used to modify commercial formulas or combined to produce unique enteral tube feeding formulas.

In the selection of a product, the resident's individual requirements and ability to tolerate carbohydrate, protein, and fat sources must be considered, as well as calorie to volume requirements. The feeding method also must be considered when choosing a formula as some formulas may require pumps for infusion.

Table 6.5 provides a description of the various types of enteral tube feeding formulas available, as well as indications for use and advantages versus disadvantages.

Table 6.5

Enteral Tube Feeding Formulas

Type	Description	Indication for use	Advantages	Disadvantages
Standard	Isotonic, low residue. Nutritionally complete. Supplies 1.0-2.0 kcal/mL. Supplies 40 g/L protein.	Maintenance to mild stress.	Inexpensive, well tolerated.	Lacks fiber.
Fiber-containing	Low osmolarity. Nutritionally complete. Supplies 1.0-2.0 kcal/mL. Supplies approximately 44 gL protein. Whole food or soy polysaccharides provide fiber source.	Maintenance to mild stress bowel dysfunction.	Provides a well-tolerated fiber source.	May cause gas, bloating, or constipation if adequate water is not supplied.
High-nitrogen	Low osmolarity. Nutritionally complete. Supplies 1.0-1.2 kcal/mL. Supplies 44-55 g/L protein.	Residents with elevated protein needs. High-stress situations.	Well tolerated. Increased protein content without increasing caloric level.	Higher protein level may require more water. May not be suitable for patients with renal insufficiency. Usually lacks fiber.
High-calorie/high-nitrogen	Nutritionally complete. Concentrated high fat content. Supplies 1.5-2.0 kcal/mL. Supplies 70-84 g/L protein.	High-stress situations for residents who have both elevated caloric and protein needs.	Concentrated formula that can be useful in residents who need to be fluid restricted.	Higher osmolarity and fat content may cause intolerance.
Elemental or chemically defined	Low residue, low fat. Predigested (may contain peptides and/or amino acids). Nutritionally complete. Supplies 1.0 kcal/mL. Supplies 40 g/L protein.	Malabsorption syndromes, fat intolerances, or high-stress situations.	Easily digested. Well tolerated (may contain significant amounts of glutamine).	Lacks fiber. May have higher osmolarity. Expensive. Only moderate level of protein.
Disease-specific	Vary in nutritional composition, depending on disease-specific recommendations.	Specific diseases (diabetes, renal failure, respiratory failure).	May help meet nutrition requirements in residents with specific problems.	May be expensive. Questionable efficiency.

INITIATING TUBE FEEDINGS

Formulas today generally are isotonic or have reasonably low osmolarity, and most residents can be started on a full strength formula successfully. When starting tube feeding it is best to advance slowly and check residuals often. If a resident is started out on a diluted formula, it is best to advance volume before strength. *Tables 6.6* and *6.7* provide sample administration schedules for continuous and intermittent feedings.

Table 6.6

Sample Administration Schedule for Formulas Having Osmolality of 300–500 mOsm/kg Water*

Continuous Schedule

Day	Time	Strength	Rate (mL/h)	Volume (mL)	Calories
1	1st 8 h	Full	50	400	400
	2nd 8 h	Full	75	600	600
	3rd 8 h	Full	100	800	800
					1800 total kcal
2	24 h	Full	100–125	2400–3000	2400–3000 total kcal

Intermittent Schedule

Day	Time	Strength	Rate (5–10 mL/min)	Volume (mL)	Calories
1	7 AM–11 PM	Full	100 mL q2h (7 AM, 9 AM)	200	200
			150 mL q2h (11 AM, 1 PM, 3 PM)	450	450
			200 mL q2h (5 PM, 7 PM, 9 PM, 11 PM)	800	800
					1450 total kcal
2	7 AM–11 PM	Full	250 mL q2h (8 feedings)	2000	2000 total kcal
			400 mL q3h (5 feedings)	2000	2000 total kcal

*If intolerance develops, use half-strength formula, or switch to a full-strength isotonic or fiber-containing diet. After tolerance to half-strength is established, continue feeding schedule until desired rate is achieved. Then switch to full strength. Do not alter rate and strength at the same time. Check gastric residuals before every intermittent feeding or every 2 to 4 h during continuous feeding. This will help avoid clogging and provide additonal water.

Note: For fiber-containing formulas, always tube feed the product at room temperature. When gravity feeding, use a size 10 French or larger tube. Smaller tubes can be used for pump delivery.

Reprinted with permission of Ross Laboratories, Columbus, OH 43216, from *Enteral Nutrition Handbook,* ©1991 Ross Laboratories.

Table 6.7

Sample Administration Schedule for Formulas Having Osmolality of >500 mOsm/kg Water

Continuous Schedule

Day	Time	Strength	Rate (mL/h)	Volume (mL)	1.0 kcal/mL	Calories 1.5 kcal/mL	2.0 kcal/mL
1	1st 8 h	½	50	400	200	300	400
	2nd 8 h	½	75	600	300	450	600
	3rd 8 h	½	100	800	400	600	800
					900	1350	1800 total kcal
2	1st 8 h	½	125	1000	500	750	1000
	2nd 8 h	Full	100–125	800–1000	400–500	1200–1500	1600–2000
	3rd 8 h	Full	100–125	800–1000	800–1000	1200–1500	1600–2000
					1700–2000	3150–3750	4200–5000 total kcal
3	24 h	Full	100–125	2400–3000	2400–3000	3600–4500	4800–6000 total kcal

Intermittent Schedule

Day	Time	Strength	Rate (mL/h)	Volume (mL)	1.0 kcal/mL	Calories 1.5 kcal/mL	2.0 kcal/mL
1	7 AM–11 PM	½	100 mL q2h (7 AM, 9 AM)	200	100	150	200
		½	150 mL q2h (11 AM, 1 PM, 3 PM)	450	225	338	450
		½	200 mL q2h (5 PM, 7 PM, 9 PM, 11 PM)	800	400	600	800
					725	1088	1450 total kcal
2	7 AM–11 PM	½	250 mL q2h (5 PM, 7 PM, 9 PM, 11 PM)	750	325	563	750
		Full	250 mL q2h (1 PM, 3 PM, 5 PM, 7 PM 9 PM, 11 PM)	1500	1500	2250	3000
					1875	2813	3750 total kcal
3	7 AM–11 PM	Full	250 mL q2h	2000	2000	3000	4000
			(8 feedings up to 400 mL q3h 5 feedings)	2000	2000	3000	4000 total kcal

*Reprinted with permission of Ross Laboratories, Columbus, OH 43216, from *Enteral Nutrition Handbook*, 1991 Ross Laboratories.

WATER REQUIREMENT

Most tube feeding formulas contain 50% to 85% water depending on the caloric density of the formula. The more calorically dense a formula is, the less water available.[1,2] When residents are on tube feeding, tube flushes are often necessary to provide additional water to prevent dehydration problems. Fluid or water is an important macronutrient that often is overlooked. An estimation of fluid requirements is approximately 1mL/kcal or 30 mL/kg body weight. When reviewing total intake of fluids the registered dietitian must take into consideration water used for irrigation, medication administration, and so forth. Overhydration can be as dangerous as dehydration.

ADMINISTRATION OF TUBE FEEDING

Tube feedings can be delivered in three different ways: bolus, continuous drip, or cyclic.

Bolus feedings are administered in 240-mL to 400-mL amounts over a short period, usually 10 minutes, or by gravity drip over 30 to 45 minutes. This is a convenient method, but can cause intolerance problems and increase the risk for aspiration. Gastric residuals should be monitored carefully in residents on bolus feeding. Bolus feedings are suitable for alert residents who want the freedom to move about the nursing facility and participate in activities.

In the *continuous drip* method, formula is slowly administered to the resident over a 24-hour period. A feeding pump is usually required, but gravity feed may be used. Continuous drip is associated with smaller residual volume and decreased possibility of pulmonary aspiration. Continuous feeding reduces complications of intolerance and reduces the risk for aspiration, but can limit mobility. Even with reduced risk for aspiration, it is still necessary to check gastric residuals routinely. The amount of time the resident is not receiving continuous feeding (eg, during therapy or baths) should be noted. If these times are an hour or more, they affect the total intake. Adjustments may be necessary to compensate for these lost calories.

With *cyclic feedings,* formula is administered during only part of the day. Feeding is often provided during the night but can be infused at specific intervals throughout the day. This is helpful for residents who only need to supplement their diet or residents who are in a transitional stage from tube feedings to an oral diet (rehabilitation therapy) or in the rehabilitation setting where residents may be in therapies during the day.

ORDERING FEEDING

The physician with the assistance of the registered dietitians, should specify:
- Formula (commercial name)
- Number of calories per 24 hours
- Volume to be given for 24 hours and strength of formula, initially, and thereafter as the tolerance is established
- Frequency of feeding per 24 hours
- Volume of water in addition to the prepared formulas
- Site of entry for tube feeding
- Method of administration (bolus, pump, drip, gravity)

MONITORING

A nutrition assessment (see Table 7.1) is completed by the registered dietitian for all enterally tube fed residents as well as others. But for the enterally tube fed resident, more specific information is needed. The questions in *Table 6.8* will help this process as well as the monitoring required. It must be remembered the caloric and protein requirements are based on estimations. For specific information about formulas for the enterally tube fed resident refer to Table 6.5. Close monitoring is required, and periodic nutrition evaluation *(Table 6.9)* is valuable in determining the effectiveness of therapy.

Table 6.8

Enteral Tube Feeding Assessment Guide

The following questions are stated to help the assessment process:

Observations:

1. Is the tube clean and does formula flow freely?
2. Is the nasal tube securely but comfortably secured on the face with skin maintained intact and without irritation?
3. Is the resident with a nasal tube for a prolonged period observed for possible complications; eg, nasal erosion, sinusitis, esophagitis, gastric ulceration, and pulmonary infection?
4. Is the skin around the gastrostomy kept clean and free from irritation or infection?
5. Is the resident fed slowly with head elevated to 45 degrees during feeding and at least 1 hour postfeeding?
6. Does the resident's mouth show signs of good mouth care?

Record review:

1. Has the tube feeding been ordered by the physician?
2. What is the order: name of formula, amount of formula, amount of calories, amount of additional water, time span over which each feeding should be accomplished?
3. a. Is the tube placement documented?
   b. How often?
4. Is the amount of tube feeding and additional water actually infused documented?
5. a. Are signs of problems documented (weight loss, diarrhea, constipation, skin condition)?
   b. How often?
   c. Have measures been taken to prevent problems and treat them if they have developed?
6. Has the nutrition assessment been documented?
7. Has periodic assessment of ability to swallow been completed and documented?

Table 6.8 (continued)

Enteral Tube Feeding Assesment Guide

If the resident can be interviewed:

1. How long have you been fed by this tube?
2. a. When was the last time you tried to eat by mouth?
   b. What happened?
3. a. How often do you receive this feeding?
   b. Is this consistent?
4. a. Do you feel comfortable and safe with all staff members who perform the feeding?
   b. If not, what happens?
5. a. Are you losing or gaining weight?
   b. What is your goal?
6. a. How often is the tube changed?
   b. Who does this?
   c. Do you feel comfortable and safe with all staff members who perform this procedure?
   d. If not, what happens?

Evaluation:

1. Is the feeding being monitored to ensure that the feeding is occurring at the ordered or appropriate rate?
2. Is the tube feeding nutritionally adequate?
3. Have attempts been made to discontinue tube feeding if indicated?
4. a. Is skin free from irritation?
   b. Is mouth care given several times daily?
5. Have changes in patient's condition been noted and addressed (weight loss, constipation, diarrhea, skin condition)?
6. Have observed problems (weight loss, constipation, diarrhea, skin condition) been coordinated with other departments and been resolved?

Adapted from *Enteral Feeding Assessment Guide.* St. Louis, Mo: Sherwood Medical; 1989.

Table 6.9

Enteral Tube Feeding Evaluation

Name _____ Room _____ DOB _____

CALORIC EVALUATION:

1. Current wt _____ (lb) Ht _____ IBW range _____ Age _____
2. BEE = Weight kcal + height kcal – age kcal
    Determine stress factor of 1.2 to 1.5
    Circle stress factors: Severe burns
                                                                Pressure sores—
    Skeletal trauma   Dehydration   Stage _____
    Draining wounds   Surgical wounds
3. Determine activity factor of
    Confined to bed 1.2 or out of bed 1.3
4. Calculate BEE × stress factor × activity factor = _____ total calories

PROTEIN EVALUATION:

1. Ideal body weight in lb _____ – 2.2 = _____ kg × 0.8 - 1 = _____ g protein needed.
    (1.2 – 1.5 if there are conditions of severe stress.)
2. Revised protein need with stress factor = _____ g protein needed.

FLUID EVALUATION:

1. Based on actual body weight over 55 years with no major cardiac or renal disease use 30 mL/kg/d.
    Body weight _____ – 2.2 = _____ kg × 30 mL = _____ mL of fluids needed per day.

LABORATORY DATA:

HCT _____ HGB _____ Alb _____ TPro _____ FBS _____
BUN _____ Na _____ K+ _____ Cl _____

SUMMARY

	ORDER GIVEN	RESIDENT'S NEEDS	RECOMMENDATION
Formula name			
Volume needed RDA			
Volume ordered			
% RDA provided			
Total calories			
Protein			
Water from formula			
Flush water*			
Method of feeding			
Volume/frequency			

*Flush water includes medication flushes.

Present tube feeding order: _____

Recommended tube feeding order: _____

RD signature _____ Date: _____

Adapted from MEP Healthcare Dietary Services, Inc, Evansville, Ind. Used by permission.

Weight change is probably the easiest indicator of successful nutrition repletion, but weight gain can also indicate fat and fluid accumulation. It is important to distinguish between fat and fluid increases versus changes in lean body mass. Some fluid accumulation is expected in the first few weeks. Weight increases of more than 2 to 3 lb per week are usually attributable to fluid.[8,9]

Besides weight, it is important to monitor protein status by checking the levels of circulating proteins. The main proteins to monitor are albumin or prealbumin and transferrin.

Albumin comprises more than 50% of the total serum proteins, and is a good indicator of nutritional status. Albumin has a long half-life and is slow to recover from nutritional stress, but it is an inexpensive way to monitor responses to nutrition therapy.[1,8,9]

Prealbumin (transthyretin) is a sensitive and reliable marker that effectively monitors the outcome of nutrition intervention. It has a half-life of two days versus albumin's 20 days; thus, it is a more sensitive marker.

Transferrin is also a more sensitive indicator of nutrition status; it has a short half-life, so it is a more reliable indicator in the acute stages of nutritional repletion. Unfortunately, prealbumin and transferrin may be more expensive and may not be readily available.[9]

Besides monitoring weight and protein status, it is also important to monitor other laboratory values, especially blood glucose, BUN, creatinine, and electrolytes in any resident receiving nutrition support therapy. For these items, protocols must be written.

With enteral tube feeding nutrition support, mechanical, GI, or metabolic complications may occur. The registered dietitian may be of tremendous assistance to nurses in identifying causes and suggesting treatment for these problems, as identified in *Table 6.10*.

Table 6.10

Enteral Tube Feeding Complications and Problem Solving

Problem	Cause	Prevention/Treatment
Mechanical complications		
Aspiration pneumonia	Delayed gastric emptying, gastroparesis	Reduce infusion rate. Select isotonic or lower-fat formula. Administer formula at room temperature. Regularly check gastric residuals.
	Gastroesophageal reflux Diminished gag reflex	Use small-bore feeding tubes to minimize compromise of lower esophageal sphincter. Keep head of bed elevated 45 degrees during and after feeding. Initially and regularly check tube placement. Feed into duodenum or jejunum, especially for high-risk patients.
Pharyngeal irritation, otitis	Prolonged intubation with large-bore NG tubes	Use small-bore feeding tubes whenever possible.
Nasolabial, esophageal, and mucosal irritation and erosion	Prolonged intubation with large-bore NG tubes Use of rubber or plastic	Use smaller-caliber feeding tubes made of biocompatible materials. Tape feeding tube properly to avoid placing pressure on the nostril. Consider gastrostomy or jejunostomy sites for long-term feeding.
Irritation and leakage at ostomy site	Drainage of digestive juices from stoma site	Attention to skin and stoma care. Use gastrostomy tubes with retention devices to maintain proper tube placement.
Tube lumen obstruction	Thickened formula residue Formation of insoluble formula-medication complexes	Irrigate feeding tube frequently with clear water. Avoid instilling medications into feeding tubes. Irrigate tubes with clear water before and after delivering medications and formula.
GI complications		
Diarrhea	Low-residue intolerance (lack of bulk)	Select fiber-supplemented formula.
	Rapid formula administration	Initiate feedings at low rate. Temporarily decrease rate.
	Hyperosmolar formula	Reduce rate of administration. Select isotonic formula or dilute formula concentration and gradually increase strength.
	Bolus feeding using syringe force	Reduce rate of administration. Select alternate method of administration.
	Hypoalbuminemia	Use elemental diet or parenteral nutrition until absorptive capacity of small intestine is restored.
	Lactose intolerance	Select lactose-free formula (most commercial formulas are lactose-free).
	Fat malabsorption	Select low-fat formula.
	Microbial contamination	Use good handling and administration techniques.
	Rapid GI transit time	Select fiber-supplemented formula.
	Prolonged antibiotic treatment or other drug therapy	Review medication profile and eliminate causative agent if possible. Repopulate normal gut flora with commerical lactobacillus.

Table 6.10 (continued)

Enteral Tube Feeding Complications and Problem Solving

Problem	Cause	Prevention/Treatment
GI complications continued		
Cramping, gas, abdominal distention	Nutrient malabsorption	Select formula that restricts offending nutrients.
	Rapid, intermittent administration of refrigerated formula	Administer formula by continuous method. Administer formula at room temperature.
	Intermittent feeding using syringe force	Reduce rate of administration. Select alternate method of administration.
Nausea and vomiting	Rapid formula administration Gastric retention	Initiate feedings at low rate and gradually advance to desired rate. Temporarily decrease rate.
		Select isotonic formula. Reduce rate of administration. Use half-strength formula. Select low-fat formula. Consider need for change in feeding route (eg, feed into duodenum or jejunum).
Constipation	Inadequate fluid intake	Supplement fluid intake.
	Insufficient bulk	Select fiber-supplemented formula.
	Inactivity	Encourage ambulation, if possible.
Metabolic complications		
Dehydration	Inadequate fluid intake or excessive losses	Supplemental fluid intake. Monitor fluid intake and output.
Overhydration	Rapid refeeding Excessive fluid intake	Reduce rate of administration, especially in patients with severe malnutriton or major organ failure. Monitor fluid intake and output and patient condition.
Hyperglycemia	Inadequate insulin production for the amount of formula being given Stress	Initiate feedings at low rate. Monitor serum and urine glucose. Use oral hypoglycemic agents or insulin if necessary.
Hypernatremia	Inadequate fluid intake or excessive losses	Supplemental fluid intake. Monitor fluid intake and output.
Hyponatremia	Inadequate intake Fluid overload Inappropriate antidiuretic hormone secretion syndrome Excessive GI fluid losses	Supplement sodium intake. Restrict fluids. Use diuretics if necessary. Replace with fluids of similar composition.
Hypophosphatemia	Aggressive refeeding of malnourished residents Insulin therapy	Monitor serum levels. Replenish phosphorus levels before refeeding.
Hypercapnia	Excessive carbohydrate loads given residents with respiratory dysfunction and CO_2 retention	Select low-carbohydrate, high-fat formula.
Hypokalemia	Aggressive refeeding of malnourished resident	Monitor serum levels. Provide adequate potassium.
Hyperkalemia	Excessive potassium intake Decreased excretion	Reduce potassium intake. Monitor serum levels.

Parenteral Administration

Parenteral nutrition is a method of nutrition support in which nutrient solutions consisting of protein (amino acids), carbohydrates (dextrose), fat (lipid), electrolytes, vitamins, and minerals are administered intravenously either: through a peripheral vein (peripheral parenteral nutrition, PPN) or through a central vein (total parenteral nutrition, TPN). Parenteral nutrition is used when the gut is not functioning or should not be used (see Table 6.4). This therapy can be used for short- and long-term support.[10]

NUTRIENT SOURCES IN PARENTERAL NUTRITION

Nutrients need to be delivered directly into the bloodstream in a form that can be assimilated at the cellular level.[11]

Protein is supplied in the form of crystalline amino acids. There are many commercially available solutions that generally contain a mix of both essential and nonessential amino acids. The concentration of amino acids can range from 3.5% to 15%, and supplies 4 kcal/g.[7] The main purpose of amino acids is to spare nitrogen or promote a positive nitrogen balance.

The fat source is supplied with either 10% or 20% lipid emulsion. This emulsion contains either soybean oil or safflower oil in combination with glycerol and emulsifiers.[7] Lipid emulsions prevent fatty acid deficiencies and provide a concentrated source of calories. These emulsions contain approximately 9 kcal/g. Most parenteral nutrition solutions contain 20% to 80% of calories from fat.[7,8]

Carbohydrates are supplied from dextrose, a six-carbon sugar that is easily assimilated into the cells for energy. Dextrose varies in concentrations ranging from 5% to 70%, and has 3.4 kcal/g. Dextrose is a major source of calories in most parenteral nutrition solutions, supplying up to 50% to 80% of total calories.

Besides dextrose, lipids, and amino acids, parenteral solutions contain vitamins and minerals. These are usually provided with commercial multiple-electrolyte solutions or parenteral vitamin supplementation based on recommendations from the the American Medical Association's Nutrition Advisory Group. To prevent clinical deficiencies multiple trace element preparations may be added to parenteral nutrition solutions.

PERIPHERAL PARENTERAL NUTRITION

A typical PPN solution supplied via peripheral venous access, may contain a combination of 3.5% amino acids, 20% dextrose, and 20% lipid emulsion.[9] The concentration of amino acids and dextrose needs to be limited in PPN to reduce problems of thrombophlebitis. As the concentration of amino acids and dextrose increases, so does the osmolarity. This produces hypertonic solutions that are irritating to peripheral veins. Luckily, lipid emulsions are isotonic, which eases the irritation.

Since both amino acids and dextrose are somewhat limited, fat supplies the majority of calories. Some PPN solutions have up to 70% to 80% fat.

Usually, PPN is intended for short-term support—mainly because the peripheral veins tolerate the concentrated hypertonic solutions poorly, making it difficult to achieve adequate calories and protein.

Routine considerations for PPN[10]:

- Fluid is usually limited to 2 to 205 L per 24 hours;
- Osmolarity should not exceed 650 to 700 mOsm/L*;
- Expected duration no greater than 7 to 10 days;
- Individual calorie and protein requirements usually cannot be met 100%;
- Lipids usually provide the major source of calories and generally should not exceed 1 g of fat per kilogram dry body weight.

Table 6.11

Estimating Osmolarity of Parenteral Nutritional Solutions

To estimate total milliosmoles per liter (mOsm/L) **calculate:**

(1)	Milliosmoles/liter from dextrose solution Final concentration of dextrose (%) × 50	_____ mOsm/L from dextrose
(2)	Milliosmoles/liter from amino acid solution Final concentration of amino acids (%) × 100	_____ mOsm/L from amino acids
(3)	Milliosmoles/liter from electrolytes (mEq Na^+/liter + mEq K^+/liter) x 2	_____ mOsm/L from electrolytes
(4)	Total estimated milliosmoles/liter Sum of mOsm/L calculated in items (1), (2) and (3)	_____ Total estimated mOsm/L of solution

Fat solutions are isotonic and do not affect osmolarity.

EXAMPLE: Estimating osmolarity of parenteral nutrition solutions:
Estimate total mOsm/L from a solution of 300 mL D_{20}, 700 mL 5.5% amino acids, 51 mEq/L Na^+ and 30 mEq/L K^+. Final concentration is 6% dextrose and 3.85% amino acids. (Actual calculations and results are shown in **bold italics**)

Calculate:

(1)	Milliosmoles/liter from dextrose solution Final concentration of dextrose(%) × 50 **(6 x 50)**	**300** mOsm/L from dextrose
(2)	Milliosmoles/liter from amino acid solution Final concentration of amino acid solution × 100 **(3.85 x 100)**	**385** mOsm/L from amino acids
(3)	Milliosmoles/liter from electrolytes (mEq Na^+/L + mEq K^+/L) × 2 **(51 + 30) x 2**	**162** mOsm/L from electrolytes
(4)	Total estimated milliosmoles/liter Sum of mOsm/L calculated in items (1), (2) and (3) **(300 + 385 + 162)**	**847** Total estimated mOsm/L of solution

Adapted from *Kansas Diet Manual*.[10] Used by permission.

---

* To estimate the total osmolarity of a parenteral nutrition solution use *Table 6.11*.

TOTAL PARENTERAL NUTRITION

This form of parenteral nutrition is prepared in a pharmacy and administered via central venous access. Access to the venous system is usually gained through the subclavian vein or the internal or external jugular vein.[8] One advantage of using TPN, is that hypertonic solutions of amino acids and dextrose can be given through a central vein; allowing adequate calories and protein to be provided.

Most central TPN solutions are a combination of 50% dextrose, 8.5% to 10% amino acids, 20% lipid emulsion, and other necessary compounds.[8]

If monitored closely, TPN can be used for long-term support. In any type of parenteral nutrition, the risk of infection is high, and careful nursing care and nutrition monitoring are essential.

Routine considerations for TPN[10]:

- Fluid levels of 30 to 50 mL per kilogram body weight are adequate for most residents but may vary depending on pathologic conditions;
- Expected duration is greater than 7 to 10 days;
- The nonstressed body tolerates 4 to 5 mg of dextrose per kilogram body weight per minute;
- A minimum of 4% of calories must be provided as fat to prevent essential fatty acid deficiency when TPN is used long term.

Most often the fat emulsion is delivered separately from the carbohydrate and protein solution (piggyback or two-bag system). Recently, fat, carbohydrate, and protein have been combined and delivered in one bag (all-in-one or three-in-one system). *Worksheets* to determine custom adult parenteral nutrition solutions with examples for each method follow. To calculate calories, carbohydrate, protein, and fat content ordered or delivered in parenteral nutrition solutions use *Table 6.12*.

Worksheet 1

Determining Parenteral Nutrition Solutions for the Piggyback System

Estimate:

(1)   Total number of calories required.   _____ kcal

(2)   Total grams of protein required.*   _____ g

Calculate:

(3)   Number of calories desired from fat.   _____ kcal from fat
       Determined as percentage of total calories.

(4)   Number of calories from protein. If protocols in your institution do not include protein   _____ kcal from
       as a source of calories then skip to item (5b); otherwise: protein
       Multiply total grams of protein in item (2) by 4.3 and go to item (5a).

(5)   Number of calories from carbohydrate (complete either 5a *or* 5b, not both).   _____ kcal from
                                                                                           carbohydrate
       (a)   Add protein calories in item (4) and fat calories in item (3) and subtract from total
              calories in item (1).

       (b)   Subtract fat calories in item (3) from total calories in item (1).

Select:

(6)   Volume and percent of dextrose (carbohydrate) solution for calories calculated in   _____ mL
       item (5).
       See Schedule A, Calories in Parenteral Nutrition Dextrose Solutions.   _____ %

(7)   Volume and percent of amino acid (protein) solution for total protein estimated in   _____ mL
       item (2).
       See Schedule B, Grams of Protein in Parenteral Nutrition Amino Acid Solutions.   _____ %

(8)   Volume and percent of lipid (fat) solution for calories calculated in item (3).   _____ mL

       See Schedule C, Average Calories and Grams of Fat Per Day with Daily or Intermit-   _____ %
       tent Administration of Lipid Solutions.

Determine:

(9)   Hourly infusion rate of dextrose-amino acid solution.   _____ mL/h
       Total mL of dextrose solution plus amino acid solution divided by 24 (h).

(10)   Hourly infusion rate of lipid solution.   _____ mL/h
       Total mL of fat solution divided by 24 (h).†

---

* Protein requirements may vary depending on the pathologic condition of the individual.

† Total volume can be delivered in less than 24 h by increasing the hourly infusion rate.

Example: Worksheet 1

Daily needs: 2000 kcal, 80 g of protein, with 25% of total calories from fat. (Actual calculations and results are shown in ***bold italics***).

Estimate:

(1)   Total number of calories required.   **2000** kcal

(2)   Total grams of protein required.   **80** g

Calculate:

(3)   Number of calories desired from fat.   **500** kcal from
     Determined as percentage of total calories.   fat
     (2000 x .25)

(4)   Number of calories from protein.   **344** kcal from
     Multiply total grams of protein in item (2) by 4.3 and go to item (5a).   protein
     (80 x 4.3)

(5)   Number of calories from carbohydrate (complete either 5a *or* 5b, not both).   **1156** kcal from
         carbohydrate

    (a)   Add protein calories in item (4) and fat calories in item (3) and subtract from total
       calories in item (1).
       2000 - (344 + 500)

Select:

(6)   Volume and percent of dextrose (carbohydrate) solution for calories calculated in   **700** mL
     item (5).   **50** %
     See Schedule A, Calories in Parenteral Nutrition Dextrose Solutions.

(7)   Volume and percent of amino acid (protein) solution for total protein estimated in item   **1000** mL
     (2).   **8** %
     See Schedule B, Grams of Protein in Parenteral Nutrition Amino Acid Solutions.

(8)   Volume and percent of lipid (fat) solution for calories calculated in item (3).   **300** mL

     See Schedule C, Average Calories and Grams of Fat Per Day with Daily or Intermit-   **20** %
     tent Administration of Lipid Solutions.

Determine:

(9)   Hourly infusion rate of dextrose-amino acid solution.   **71** mL/h
     Total mL of dextrose solution plus amino acid solution divided by 24 (h).
     (700 + 1000) ÷ 24

(10)   Hourly infusion rate of lipid solution.   **12.5** mL/h
     Total mL of fat solution divided by 24 (h).*   (6 d/wk)
     (300 ÷ 24)

---

* Total volume can be delivered in less than 24 h by increasing the hourly infusion rate.

Schedule A: Calories in Parenteral Nutrition Dextrose Solutions

Calories	Volume mL	% Dextrose solution	Calories	Volume mL	% Dextrose solution	Calories	Volume mL	% Dextrose solution
17	100	5	170	100	50	680	1000	20
34	200	5	204	600	10	680	400	50
34	100	10	204	300	20	714	300	70
51	300	5	238	700	10	850	500	50
68	400	5	238	100	70	952	400	70
68	200	10	272	800	10	1020	600	50
68	100	20	272	400	20	1190	700	50
85	500	5	306	900	10	1190	500	70
102	600	5	340	1000	10	1360	800	50
102	300	10	340	500	20	1428	600	70
119	700	5	340	200	50	1530	900	50
136	800	5	408	600	20	1666	700	70
136	400	10	476	700	20	1700	1000	50
136	200	20	476	200	70	1904	800	70
153	900	5	510	300	50	2142	900	70
170	1000	5	544	800	20	2380	1000	70
170	500	10	612	900	20			

How to use this schedule:

1. Match calories needed from dextrose solution with nearest value listed under the column *Calories*.

2. Read corresponding columns to determine volume and percent dextrose solution. Depending on volume and percent of solution more than one choice may be shown. Choice of solution to meet individual needs may vary according to packaging and/or strength of solutions available and procedures of the health care facility.

Schedule B: Grams of Protein in Parenteral Nutrition Amino Acid Solutions

Grams of protein	Volume mL	% Amino acid solution	Grams of protein	Volume mL	% Amino acid solution	Grams of protein	Volume mL	% Amino acid solution
3.5	100	3.5	24.0	300	8.0	45.0	900	5.0
5.0	100	5.0	24.5	700	3.5	45.9	900	5.1
5.1	100	5.1	25.0	500	5.0	48.0	600	8.0
5.5	100	5.5	25.5	500	5.1	49.0	700	7.0
7.0	200	3.5	25.5	300	8.5	49.5	900	5.5
7.0	100	7.0	27.5	500	5.5	50.0	1000	5.0
8.0	100	8.0	28.0	800	3.5	50.0	500	10.0
8.5	100	8.5	28.0	400	7.0	51.0	1000	5.1
10.0	200	5.0	30.0	600	5.0	51.0	600	8.5
10.0	100	10.0	30.0	300	10.0	55.0	1000	5.5
10.2	200	5.1	30.6	600	5.1	56.0	800	7.0
10.5	300	3.5	31.5	900	3.5	56.0	700	8.0
11.0	200	5.5	32.0	400	8.0	59.5	700	8.5
14.0	400	3.5	33.0	600	5.5	60.0	600	10.0
14.0	200	7.0	34.0	400	8.5	63.0	900	7.0
15.0	300	5.0	35.0	700	5.0	64.0	800	8.0
15.3	300	5.1	35.0	1000	3.5	68.0	800	8.5
16.0	200	8.0	35.0	500	7.0	70.0	1000	7.0
16.5	300	5.5	35.7	700	5.1	70.0	700	10.0
17.0	200	8.5	38.5	700	5.5	72.0	900	8.0
17.5	500	3.5	40.0	800	5.0	76.5	900	8.5
20.0	400	5.0	40.0	500	8.0	80.0	1000	8.0
20.0	200	10.0	40.0	400	10.0	80.0	800	10.0
20.4	400	5.1	40.8	800	5.1	85.0	1000	8.5
21.0	600	3.5	42.0	600	7.0	90.0	900	10.0
21.0	300	7.0	42.5	500	8.5	100.0	1000	10.0
22.0	400	5.5	44.0	800	5.5			

How to use this schedule:

1. Match protein needed from amino acid solution with nearest value listed under the column *Grams of protein*.

2. Read corresponding columns to determine volume and percent of amino acid solution. Depending on the volume and percent of solution more than one choice may be shown. Choice of solution to meet individual needs may vary according to packaging and/or strength of solutions available and procedures of the health care facility.

Schedule C: Average Calories and Grams of Fat Per Day with Daily or Intermittent Administration of Lipid Solutions

Calories avg/d	% Fat	Frequency (per wk)	Volume mL	Fat grams avg/d	Calories avg/d	% Fat	Frequency (per wk)	Volume mL	Fat grams avg/d
16	10	1	100	1.4	200	20	7	100	20.0
29	20	1	100	2.9	220	10	7	200	20.0
31	10	1	200	2.9	229	20	2	400	22.9
31	10	2	100	2.9	229	20	4	200	22.9
47	10	1	300	4.3	236	10	3	500	21.4
47	10	3	100	4.3	236	10	5	300	21.4
57	20	1	200	5.7	251	10	4	400	22.9
57	20	2	100	5.7	257	20	3	300	25.7
63	10	1	400	5.7	283	10	6	300	25.7
63	10	2	200	5.7	286	20	2	500	28.6
63	10	4	100	5.7	286	20	5	200	28.6
79	10	1	500	7.1	314	10	4	500	28.6
79	10	5	100	7.1	314	10	5	400	28.6
86	20	1	300	8.6	330	10	7	300	30.0
86	20	3	100	8.6	343	20	3	400	34.3
94	10	2	300	8.6	343	20	4	300	34.3
94	10	3	200	8.6	343	20	6	200	34.3
94	10	6	100	8.6	377	10	6	400	34.3
110	10	7	100	10.0	393	10	5	500	35.7
114	20	1	400	11.4	400	20	7	200	40.0
114	20	2	200	11.4	429	20	3	500	42.9
114	20	4	100	11.4	429	20	5	300	42.9
126	10	2	400	11.4	440	10	7	400	40.0
126	10	4	200	11.4	457	20	4	400	45.7
141	10	3	300	12.9	471	10	6	500	42.9
143	20	1	500	14.3	514	20	6	300	51.4
143	20	5	100	14.3	550	10	7	500	50.0
157	10	2	500	14.3	571	20	4	500	57.1
157	10	5	200	14.3	571	20	5	400	57.1
171	20	2	300	17.1	600	20	7	300	60.0
171	20	3	200	17.1	686	20	6	400	68.6
171	20	6	100	17.1	714	20	5	500	71.4
189	10	3	400	17.1	800	20	7	400	80.0
189	10	4	300	17.1	857	20	6	500	85.7
189	10	6	200	17.1	1000	20	7	500	100.0

How to use this schedule:

1. Match calories needed from lipid solution with nearest value listed under the column *Calories. avg/d.*

2. Read corresponding columns to determine percent fat, frequency of delivery (per week), and volume. Depending on percent, volume and frequency of delivery of solution more than one choice may be shown. Choice of solution to meet individual needs may vary according to packaging and/or strength of solutions available and procedures of the health care facility.

Adapted from *Kansas Diet Manual.*[10] Used by permission.

Worksheet 2
Determining Parenteral Nutrition Solutions
for the All-in-One System

Estimate:

(1) Total number of calories required.   _____ kcal

(2) Determine total fluid requirement in liters per day.   _____ L of fluid
                                                                                     per day

(3) Total grams of protein required.   _____ g protein

Calculate:

(4) Number of calories from protein.   _____ kcal from
     Multiply total grams of protein in item (3) by 4.3.   protein

(5) Number of calories from fat.   _____ kcal from
     Determined as percentage of total calories.   fat

(6) Number of calories from carbohydrate.   _____ kcal from
     Add protein calories in item (4) and fat calories in item (5) and subtract from total   carbohydrate
     calories in item (1).

(7) Number of grams of carbohydrate.   _____ g of
     Divide carbohydrate calories in item (6) by 3.4.   carbohydrate

Determine:

(8) Concentration of amino acids (g/L).   _____ g amino
     Divide total grams of protein from item (3) by fluid requirement in item (2). Generally   acid/L
     rounded to nearest 10 g but for more exact formula round to nearest 5 g.

(9) Concentration of carbohydrate (g/L).   _____ g of
     Divide total grams of carbohydrate in item (7) by total fluid requirement in item (2).   carbohydrate/L
     Round to nearest standard concentration* or for more exact concentration record exact
     value.

(10) Milliliters (mL) of 20% fat solution per liter.   _____ mL of fat/L
     (a) For total mL of fat solution divide fat calories in item (5) by 2.

     (b) Divide total mL of fat solution from item (10a) by total fluid requirement in item (2)
     for mL of fat/L.

(11) Hourly infusion rate of dextrose–amino acid–fat solution.   _____ mL/h
     Multiply total fluid requirement in item (2) by 1000 and divide by 24 (h).

---

* Standard concentrations in g/L are : 50, 100, 150, 200, and 250.

Example: Worksheet 2

Daily needs: 2000 kcal, 80 g of protein, 25% of total calories from fat, and 2.5 L of fluid. (Actual calculations and results are shown in ***bold italics***).

Estimate:

(1) Total number of calories required.   ***2000*** kcal

(2) Determine total fluid requirement in liters per day.   ***2.5*** L of fluid per day

(3) Total grams of protein required.   ***80*** g protein

Calculate:

(4) Number of calories from protein.
    Multiply total grams of protein in item (3) by 4.3.
    (80 x 4.3)   ***344*** kcal from protein

(5) Number of calories from fat.
    Determined as percentage of total calories.
    (2000 x .25)   ***500*** kcal from fat

(6) Number of calories from carbohydrate.
    Add protein calories in item (4) and fat calories in item (5) and subtract from total calories in item (1).
    2000 - (344 + 500)   ***1156*** kcal from carbohydrate

(7) Number of grams of carbohydrate.
    Divide carbohydrate calories in item (6) by 3.4.
    (1156 ÷ 3.4)   ***340*** g of carbohydrate

Determine:

(8) Concentration of amino acids (g/L).
    Divide total grams of protein from item (3) by total fluid requirement in item (2).
    (80 ÷ 2.5)   ***30*** g amino acid/L

(9) Concentration of carbohydrate (g/L).
    Divide total grams of carbohydrate in item (7) by total fluid requirement in item (2).
    (340 ÷ 2.5)   ***150*** g of carbohydrate/L

(10) Milliliters (mL) of 20% fat solution per liter.   ***100*** mL of fat/L
    (a) For total mL of fat solution divide fat calories in item (5) by 2.
    (500 ÷ 2) = 250

    (b) Divide total mL of fat solution from item (10a) by total fluid requirement in item (2) for mL of fat/L.
    (250 ÷ 2.5)

(11) Hourly infusion rate of dextrose-amino acid-fat solution.   ***104*** mL/h
    Multiply total fluid requirement in item (2) by 1000 and divide by 24 (h).
    (2.5 x 1000) ÷ 24

Adapted from *Kansas Diet Manual*.[10] Used by permission.

Table 6.12
Calculating Carbohydrate, Protein, and Fat in Commonly Used Parenteral Nutrition Solutions

Parenteral Nutrition Solutions: Calculation for Carbohydrate*

% Dextrose	Volume of Dextrose Solution									
	100	200	300	400	500	600	700	800	900	1000
5										0.05
5.5										0.055
10	0.01	0.02	0.03	0.04	0.05	0.06	0.07	0.08	0.09	0.10
20	0.02	0.04	0.06	0.08	0.10	0.12	0.14	0.16	0.18	0.20
50	0.05	0.10	0.15	0.20	0.25	0.30	0.35	0.40	0.45	0.50
70	0.07	0.14	0.21	0.28	0.35	0.42	0.49	0.56	0.63	0.70

How to use this chart:

1. Check parenteral nutrition order sheet in the medical record to determine percentage and volume of dextrose in nutrition solution.
2. Find the percentage of dextrose/L of solution by reading down the left side vertical column on the calculation chart.
3. Find the volume of dextrose/L of solution by reading across the top horizontal row on the calculation chart.
4. Find the grid on the chart where these two lines intersect.
5. Multiply total volume of solution delivered by the factor located in the grid. The product equals grams of carbohydrate delivered.
6. To determine calories delivered, multiply grams of carbohydrate by 3.4.

Parenteral Nutrition Solutions: Calculation for Protein*

% Amino Acid Solution	Volume of Amino Acid Solution									
	100	200	300	400	500	600	700	800	900	1000
5.1	0.0051	0.010	0.015	0.020	0.025	0.030	0.035	0.040	0.045	0.051
5.5	0.0055	0.011	0.016	0.022	0.027	0.033	0.038	0.044	0.049	0.055
7	0.007	0.014	0.021	0.028	0.035	0.042	0.049	0.056	0.063	0.070
8	0.008	0.016	0.024	0.032	0.040	0.048	0.056	0.064	0.072	0.080
8.5	0.0085	0.017	0.025	0.034	0.042	0.051	0.059	0.068	0.076	0.085
10	0.01	0.02	0.03	0.04	0.05	0.06	0.07	0.08	0.09	0.10

How to use this chart:

1. Check parenteral nutrition order sheet in the medical record to determine percentage and volume of amino acids in nutrition solution.
2. Find the percentage of amino acids/L of solution by reading down the left side vertical column on the calculation chart.
3. Find the volume of amino acids/L of solution by reading across the top horizontal row on the calculation chart.
4. Find the grid on the chart where these two lines intersect.
5. Multiply total volume of solution delivered by the factor located in the grid. The product equals grams of protein infused.
6. To determine calories delivered multiply grams of protein by 4.3.

Parenteral Nutrition Solutions: Calculation for Fat*

% Lipid	Grams of Fat/mL	Calories/mL†
10	0.1	1.1
20	0.2	2.0

How to use this chart:

1. Determine percentage and volume of lipid solution ordered.
2. To determine grams of fat, multiply total volume of lipid solution delivered by grams of fat/mL.
3. To determine calories delivered, multiply total volume of lipid solution delivered by calories/mL.

* Reference: Campbell SM, ed. *Practical Guide to Nutritional Care.* University of Alabama Hospital; 1984:81–82.

† Represents the calories from both fat and the emulsifying agents.

Note: Calories derived from amino acid solutions may or may not be calculated as part of the energy source in parenteral nutrition solutions.

Adapted from *Kansas Diet Manual.*[10] Used by permission.

References

1. Rombeau JL, Caldwell MD. *Clinical Nutrition Enteral and Tube Feeding.* 2nd ed. Philadelphia, Pa: WB Saunders Co; 1990.
2. Chernoff R, Lipschitz DA. Enteral feeding and the geriatric patient. In: Rombeau JL, Caldwell MD. *Clinical Nutrition Enteral and Tube Feeding.* 2nd ed. Philadelphia, Pa: WB Saunders Co; 1990.
3. *Pocket Resource for Nutritional Assessment.* Chicago, Ill: Consultant Dietitians in Health Care Facilities Dietetic Practice Group; 1990.
4. Campbell S, Geraghty M, Behr S. *Enteral Nutrition Handbook.* Columbus, Ohio: Ross Laboratories; 1991.
5. Alpers DH, Clouse RE, Stenson WF. *Manual of Nutritional Therapeutics.* 2nd ed. Boston, Mass: Little Brown and Co; 1990.
6. Shrounts EP, ed. *Nutrition Support Dietetics Core Curriculum.* Silver Spring, Md: American Society of Parenteral and Enteral Nutrition; 1989.
7. Chicago Dietetic Association, South Suburban Dietetic Association. *Manual of Clinical Dietetics.* Chicago, Ill: The American Dietetic Association; 1988.
8. American Society for Parenteral and Enteral Nutrition. Standards for nutrition support for residents for long-term care facilities. *Nutr Clin Pract.* 1989;4:148–153.
9. Thomas DR, Verdery RB, Gardner L, Kant A, et al. A prospective study of outcome from protein energy malnutrition in nursing home residents. *JPEN J Parenter Enteral Nutr* 1991;15:400–404.
10. Parenteral nutrition. In: *Kansas Diet Manual.* Kansas City, Kan: Kansas Dietetic Association; 1992.
11. Pillar B, Perry S. Evaluating total parenteral nutrition: final report and statement of the Technology Assessment and Practice Guidelines forum. *Nutrition.* 1990;6:314–318.

7. Nutrition Assessment

Resident Interview—Diet History

Anthropometry

Calories and Fluid

Reassessments

7. NUTRITION ASSESSMENT

A nutrition assessment is the systematic method of gathering data to determine a resident's current nutritional status and to develop a plan of care.

An initial nutrition assessment identifies the strengths and weaknesses that contribute to the nutritional status of the resident and identifies residents at nutritional risk. The assessment form *(Table 7.1)* guides the dietetic technician, dietary manager, and registered dietitian in collecting information for developing a plan of care. The assessment provides the information to complete the minimum data set (MDS) for nursing facility resident assessment and care screening.

Table 7.1

Nutrition Assessment Form

Name _____   Admission date _____ Room _____

DOB _____ Ht _____ Sex M/F   Diet order _____

Wt _____ lb ÷ 2.2 = _____ kg   Food allergies _____

Wrist circumference _____   Supplement order _____

Frame size: sm   med   lg   Diagnosis _____

Ideal body wt range _____ + _____ = _____   _____
                    − 2 = desirable body wt

Recent weight loss yes / no _____ lb _____ %   Physician _____

Explain _____

Degree of self-help

_____ Independent

_____ Needs some assistance
          (butter bread, etc)

_____ Needs supervision

_____ Needs to be fed

_____ Needs self-help feeding device;
          Type: _____

_____ Needs firm encouragement to
          eat or complete meal

_____ Enteral feeding

_____ Parenteral/IV

_____ Syringe fed

Psychosocial well-being

(Check all that apply)

_____ Eats in dining room

_____ Eats in rehab dining room

_____ Eats in room by choice

_____ Eats out occasionally

Mobility

_____ Cane/walker

_____ Brace

_____ Wheelchair

_____ Geri chair

_____ Independent

Skin Condition

_____ Dry

_____ Fragile

_____ Pressure ulcer

          _____ stage

_____ Number of pressure ulcers

_____ No problems

Communication/barriers

_____ Hearing aid

_____ Signs/gestures

_____ Writes to express needs

_____ Adequate; no problems

Cognitive pattern

_____ Resident alert,
          information reliable

_____ Resident somewhat confused;
          check information with family
          and/or nursing

_____ Resident unable to relate
          reliable information; all
          information obtained from
          family/nursing

Vision

_____ Glasses _____ Blind

_____ Impaired

_____ Side vision problem; leaves
          food on one side of plate

_____ Adequate; no problems

Oral status

_____ Dentures

          _____ Full   _____ Partial

          _____ Loose   _____ Will not wear

_____ Few teeth   _____ Poor cond

_____ Edentulous

_____ Pockets food

_____ Difficulty chewing

_____ Difficulty swallowing

_____ Mouth pain

_____ Own teeth; good condition

_____ Abnormal tongue

Other factors

_____ Nausea/vomiting

_____ Constipation

_____ Diarrhea

_____ Hiatal hernia

_____ Gastric distress

_____ No problems

Fluid/hydration

_____ Hydrated

_____ Edema

_____ Dehydrated

_____ Ascites

Estimated nutrition needs:

Calories _____ Protein (g) _____

Fluids (mL) _____

Nutrition intervention:

_____ Yes   _____ No

_____ Increased portions

_____ Small portions

_____ Supplement

_____ Calories/protein

_____ Menu enrichment

_____ Vitamins/minerals

_____ Other

Describe _____

_____

Most meals

_____ Leaves 25% of food on plate

_____ % food consumed

_____ Fluid taken (mL)

_____ Accepts all food groups

          _____ Groups omitted

Table 7.1 (continued)

Nutrition Assessment Form

Laboratory values
(Specify)

BUN _____   Albumin _____   Hemoglobin _____

Cholesterol _____   Total protein _____   Hematocrit _____

Glucose _____   Sodium _____   Other _____

Prealbumin _____   Potassium _____   Other _____

Medications with nutrition implication:
Medication review   Side effects   Comments
(nutritionally pertinent)

	Altered taste	Anorexia	Hunger	Thirst	Diarrhea	Constipation	Nausea/vomiting	Flatulence	Dyspepsia	Abdominal pain	Wt variances	Dry mouth	Sore tongue	Confusion	Headache	Fatigue/weakness	Glucose variances	

Summary _____

_____

Completion date: _____ MDS _____ Triggers _____ RAP summary

Signature of dietetic technician/dietary manager   Date

Signature of registered dietitian   Date

Adapted from MEP Healthcare Dietary Services, Inc, Evansville, Ind. Reprinted with permission.

The assessment should include these major parameters:

- Nutritional history—cultural and ethnic preferences, food allergies or intolerance
- Food and fluid intake—observation of quantity and quality of intake
- Evaluation of physical conditions—including cognitive pattern, vision, physical functioning, oral/dental, oral/nutritional status, skin condition
- Anthropometrics—including recent weight variance
- Caloric and fluid requirements
- Laboratory indicators (see chapter 6)
- Food-medication interactions (see chapter 6)
- Enteral or parenteral feedings (see chapter 6)

Input should be encouraged from the nursing personnel, admissions coordinator, social worker, occupational therapist, speech language pathologist, and activities coordinator, as well as family. The resident and family provide information related to the resident's physical status prior to admission, ie, diagnosis, prior living arrangements, major surgery, or fractures. Before conducting an interview, the dietetic technician, dietary manager, or registered dietitian collects basic facts about the resident, such as the diet order, diagnosis, height, weight, dental status, ability to feed self, special problems, food and fluid intake, and procedures such as chemotherapy or dialysis.

Staff members' documentation of the resident's intake of foods and fluids is an essential part of the assessment process. The MDS requires a minimum of 3 days' observation prior to its completion. Observation of the resident's intake of meals for 3 days to determine consumption of fluids and foods is an essential part of the assessment process. *Table 7.2*, the Food Acceptance Record, is included to help staff members evaluate the resident's food and fluid consumption. Recording the percentage of food consumed by food group may reveal a potential nutritional deficiency (eg, the resident who refuses meat and protein foods and has pressure ulcers). Insufficient fluid intake can trigger dehydration. The Food Acceptance Record alerts the registered dietitian to the factors that contributed to reduced intake. Interviews of the resident and family will also contribute important information.

Table 7.2   Food Acceptance Record

		1	2	3	4	5	6	7	8	9	10	11	12	13	14	15	16	17	18	19	20	21	22	23	24	25	26	27	28	29	30	31
B R E A K F A S T	Milk (oz)																															
	Meat/egg cheese/entree																															
	Vegetable fruit/juice																															
	Bread/grain rice/pasta																															
	Beverage (oz)																															
	Initials																															
D I N N E R	Milk (oz)																															
	Meat/egg cheese/entree																															
	Vegetable fruit/juice																															
	Bread/grain rice/pasta																															
	Beverage (oz)																															
	Initials																															
S U P P E R	Milk (oz)																															
	Meat/egg cheese/entree																															
	Vegetable fruit/juice																															
	Bread/grain rice/pasta																															
	Beverage (oz)																															
	Initials																															
S U P P L E M E N T	Midmorning																															
	Midafternoon																															
	HS																															

Resident food intake

Guidelines for determining meal percentages. Follow schedule outlined below:

Milk or juice	10%	Milk	10%
Meat	30%	Meat or egg	30%
Vegetable or salad	10%	Juice	10%
Bread	10%	Cereal	30%
Potato or substitute	20%	Toast or substitute	20%
Dessert	20%		

An item is eaten less than 1/4 of amount served—no credit shall be given.
An item is eaten more than 3/4 of amount served—full credit shall be given.
Add all item percentages to determine total meal intake.

Fluid intake
Small glass — 120 mL/4 oz
Large glass — 240 mL/8 oz
Cup — 180 mL/6 oz

Dish of ice cream or gelatin
dessert — 120 mL/4 oz
Bowl of soup — 180 mL/6 oz

NAME _____ Month/year _____

Adapted from MEP Healthcare Dietary Services, Inc, Evansville, Ind. Reprinted with permission.

Resident Interview—Diet History

Interviewing an elderly resident requires skill, sensitivity, and patience. Knock before entering the room; introduce yourself and the department you represent and explain the purpose of the visit. Address residents formally (Mrs Jones, Mr Smith) to indicate respect for them as adults able to make their own decisions. Be attentive and allow time for responses; answer questions as they arise.

The interview provides the opportunity to discover food preferences. Mealtime is the highlight of the day in nursing facilities, and residents' satisfaction at mealtime is a link to their nutritional well-being. Residents' rights are an important component of the Omnibus Budget Reconciliation Act (OBRA) survey process, and a resident who consumes a balanced diet reduces the risk of nutritional complications.

Follow printed forms such as Diet History *(Table 7.3)* and Resident Food Preference *(Table 7.4)* for the interview. Review each item, paying attention to food groups that the resident dislikes and that can result in a deficiency, such as calcium.

Table 7.3

Diet History

Name _____ Room No. _____ Diet _____

Date of birth _____ Adm. Date _____ Adm Wt _____ Dr. _____

DO YOU HAVE FOOD ALLERGIES?   yes/no   If yes, specify _____

Beverage				Bread		Breakfast Cereal	
Breakfast	C	T	M _____	White _____		Hot _____	
Dinner	C	T	M _____	Wheat _____		Cold _____	
Supper	C	T	M _____	Either _____		Either _____	
				None _____		None _____	

Circle size of portion preferred: Large   Regular   Small

Do you wear glasses? or have difficulty seeing?	yes/no	If yes, specify _____
Do you wear dentures?	yes/no	upper lower both
Do you have difficulty chewing meats?	yes/no	If yes, will you eat ground? yes/no
Do you have difficulty chewing raw fruits and vegetables?	yes/no	
Do you require pureed foods?	yes/no	
Do you have difficulty cutting meats?	yes/no	
Do you have difficulty feeding yourself	yes/no	
Do you use an assistive device to help you eat?	yes/no	
Do you have difficulty swallowing?	yes/no	If yes, specify _____
Do you avoid spicy food?	yes/no	
Do you avoid nuts, seeds and/or hulls?	yes/no	
Do you have difficulty with "tomatoey" foods? i.e. spaghetti	yes/no	
Do you eat fried foods?	yes/no	
Do you drink water with your meal?	yes/no	
Do you drink water through the day?	yes/no	
Do you drink prune juice or eat prunes every morning?	yes/no	
Do you drink citrus juices, i,e, orange?	yes/no	
Do you have food brought to you from outside sources?	yes/no	
Do you get hungry between meals	yes/no	
Do you get hungry before bed at night?	yes/no	
Do you understand your diet?	yes/no	
Do you have a good appetite?	yes/no	If no, specify _____

Do you eat: Likes
                                                                     _____
_____ eggs, type of _____   _____
_____ beef   _____ raw fruit   _____
_____ pork   _____ citrus fruits   Dislikes
_____ fish   _____ other fruits   _____
_____ liver   _____
_____ poultry   _____
_____ cheese   _____
_____ cottage cheese   Comments
_____ milk If no, specify why _____   _____
_____ gravy   _____
_____ sauces, i.e., cheese, hollandaise   _____
_____ broccoli, cauliflower   _____
_____ raw vegetable salads, i.e., lettuce, coleslaw   _____
_____ other vegetables, i.e., cooked carrots, peas, corn, etc.   _____

Signature _____   Updated _____

Date: _____   _____

From C.L. Gerwick and Associates Inc, Overland Park, Kan. 1992. Reprinted with permission.

Table 7.4

Resident Food Preference

Milk	Yes	No
Sweet	___	___
Buttermilk	___	___
Chocolate	___	___

Fruits		
Apples	___	___
Applesauce	___	___
Apricots	___	___
Grapefruit	___	___
Pears	___	___
Pineapple	___	___
Plums	___	___
Prunes/juice	___	___
Peaches	___	___
Bananas	___	___
Fruit cocktail	___	___
Watermelon	___	___
Cantaloupe	___	___
Oranges	___	___
Orange juice	___	___

Breads/cereal		
Corn flakes	___	___
Bran flakes	___	___
Oatmeal	___	___
Rice	___	___
Cream of wheat	___	___
Spaghetti	___	___
Macaroni	___	___
Biscuits	___	___
Cornbread	___	___
Pancakes/ French toast	___	___

Soups		
Chili	___	___
Potato	___	___
Tomato	___	___

Soups	Yes	No
Vegetable	___	___
Beef	___	___
Bean	___	___
Other	___	___

Beverages		
Hot tea	___	___
Coffee	___	___
Iced tea	___	___

Breakfast		
Cereal of choice	___	___
Egg, favorite style	___	___
Juice or fruit	___	___

Vegetables		
Asparagus	___	___
Beets	___	___
Broccoli	___	___
Brussels sprouts	___	___
Black-eyed peas	___	___
Cabbage	___	___
Carrots	___	___
Cauliflower	___	___
Corn	___	___
Green beans	___	___
Lima beans	___	___
Navy beans	___	___
Onions	___	___
Peas	___	___
Potatoes	___	___
Pumpkin	___	___
Sauerkraut	___	___
Squash	___	___
Spinach	___	___

Vegetables	Yes	No
Tomatoes (canned)	___	___
(fresh)	___	___
Yams/sweet potatoes	___	___

Salads		
Lettuce	___	___
Coleslaw	___	___
Cottage cheese	___	___
Cucumbers	___	___
American cheese	___	___
Gelatin	___	___
Cranberry sauce	___	___
Macaroni salad	___	___
Potato chips	___	___
Pea salad	___	___
Mixed-bean salad	___	___

Meats		
Eggs	___	___
Bacon	___	___
Sausage	___	___
Weiners	___	___
Chicken (baked)	___	___
(fried)	___	___
Turkey	___	___
Pork chop	___	___
Roast beef	___	___
Hamburger	___	___
Meatloaf	___	___
Fish (baked)	___	___
(fried)	___	___
Tuna	___	___
Liver	___	___
Casseroles	___	___
Other:	___	___

Name _____   Room number _____

From MEP Healthcare Dietary Services Inc, Evansville, Ind. Reprinted by permission.

Explain the type of diet that the physician prescribed, the mealtime, and the type of food served at mealtime, whether the main meal is at noon or in the evening. Residents may not be familiar with eating four or five meals, as is the pattern in some facilities, and they should have the flexibility to choose mealtimes based on the policy of the facility. A continental breakfast might satisfy the resident who does not rise early. Point out the location of the dining room and where the menus are posted.

During the interview, it is important to establish a positive relationship with the resident. The mutual goal is to maintain or improve the quality of life for the resident.

To achieve the highest level of functioning, a resident must be able to eat independently. The registered dietitian should identify any physical barriers that interfere with the resident's ability to eat without assistance. Using the MDS as a guide, observe the resident's strengths and weaknesses in each section.

Cognitive Patterns

Is the resident alert, able to voice food preferences, and remember mealtimes? Has the resident's thought process altered the ability to eat independently? A resident may be forgetful but still have the ability to eat independently if prompted by the staff. Does the resident display indications of paranoia related to food or meal service?

Communication and Hearing Patterns

Although the talkative resident seems eager to communicate, the nonverbal resident often requires more attention from the interviewer. Ample time for response must be given. Silence can be a skillful interview technique; allow residents time to collect their thoughts. Encourage communication by using short interjections such as "I see," "yes," and "go on." It may be necessary to repeat the question if the resident seems confused or obviously does not understand. Be aware of physical impairments such as a speech disorder or hearing loss that may affect the interview.

Because hearing loss is common in elderly residents, the interviewer must be aware of individual sounds that compose the key words in a sentence. "Voiceless" sounds—those made with the lips, tongue, and teeth only—may sound distorted or may not be heard at all. Examples of voiceless sounds are *p* as in "pill" or "pork"; *f* as in "fruit" or "phone"; *t* as in "two" or "toast"; *k* as in "cup" or "could"; *h* as in "ham" or "house"; *s* as in "citrus" or "sip"; *sh* as in "fish" or "shoe"; *ch* as in "church" or "cheese." "Did you take your pill?" may be heard by the resident as "Did you say you're ill?" and answered by, "Thank you, I feel much better today."

To facilitate communication with a resident who has some hearing loss:
- Obtain resident's attention;
- Look directly at the resident;

- Speak slowly, clearly, and normally in a natural tone of voice;
- Make sure the resident is not looking into direct sunlight or other bright light; the resident may be unable to see your face if you stand at a window;
- Use short, meaningful sentences and appropriate gestures;
- Write directions, proper names, and numbers for the resident as you speak.

Vision Patterns

Visual impairments can contribute to decreased food intake at meals. Interviewers should alert staff members to give verbal cues for meal placement, using the clock method. Decreased peripheral vision requires moving the food into the line of sight. Ask the resident (not family or friends) how much help is needed. For example: Should meat be cut? Should bread be buttered? Should the location of the food on the plate be described? Many persons who have lost their sight have worked out solutions to locating their food and do not like being treated like children.

Physical Functioning

Two measures of dependence are commonly employed to assess nutritional status. Activities of daily living (ADL) measure the very basic daily care activities such as feeding, continence, walking, toileting, dressing, and bathing. The second measure, instrumental activities of daily living (IADL) measure management activities important to independent living; eg, using the telephone, handling own finances, keeping room in order, shopping for personal items, remembering to take medication, remembering mealtime and dining room location. Impairment in ADLs and IADLs can be indicative of a lack of ability to perform those activities that support good nutritional status. Thus, a general indication of functional status can help in determining the degree of nutritional risk. Until more sensitive indicators for eating dependency are developed, inability to perform one or more ADLs or IADLs related to nutrition care may be a warning of increased risk.

Determine whether the resident needs limited, extensive, or no assistance with meals and snacks. Residents commonly require some assistance in opening condiment packets or milk containers, since these procedures involve hand-eye coordination. Physical concerns that affect eating are paralysis, lack of hand dexterity, or contracture to hands, which affects the ability to handle feeding utensils. Paralysis can result in chewing or swallowing problems that require modifying the texture of the food. Smoking may alter taste and smell, which impair oral intake and decrease meal satisfaction. Some residents have the stamina to feed themselves breakfast and the noon meal but tire before the evening meal. Refer to chapter 8 for additional information.

Oral and Dental Status

Dental problems such as loose-fitting dentures may require the assistance of the social service director to contact the dentist and correct the problem. Carefully observe the resident who is endentulous, has poor teeth, or has ill-fitting dentures before recommending a consistency alteration.

Lesions in the mouth and sore or bleeding gums both affect oral intake and are an automatic trigger on the MDS, requiring the attention of the registered dietitian. Oral status includes evaluation of texture modification. A resident with loose or ill-fitting dentures may require a mechanically altered diet (eg, chopped or ground meat). A resident who has difficulty swallowing may also require texture modification. The registered dietitian, speech language pathologist, and occupational therapist should work as a team in evaluating the need for thickened liquids, texture modifications, and self-help feeding devices.

Skin Condition

Observe the resident's skin condition including signs of dehydration, edema, and/or ascites. These symptoms may signal protein deficiency, or renal or hepatic disease; all have potential nutritional significance. Loose skin may be evidence of weight loss, and the interviewer should question the resident about his or her usual weight. Make a visual scan for dry, flaky skin, which can relate to dehydration or for a non-healing wound, purpura, or bruises. Refer to *Table 7.5*, Physical Signs of Malnutrition, to help identify the problems.

Table 7.5

Physical Signs of Malnutrition

Signs	Possible causes
Hair	
Dull, dry; lack of natural shine	Protein-energy deficiency
Thin, sparse; loss of curl	Zinc deficiency
Color changes; depigmentation; easily plucked	Other nutrient deficiencies: manganese, copper
Eyes	
Small, yellowish lumps around eyes	Hyperlipidemia
White rings around both eyes	
Pale eye membranes	Vitamin B_{12}, folacin, and/or iron deficiency
Night blindness, dry membranes, dull or soft cornea	Vitamin A, zinc deficiency
Redness and fissures of eyelid corners	Niacin deficiency
Angular inflammation of eyelids	Riboflavin deficiency
Ring of fine blood vessels around cornea	General poor nutrition
Lips	
Redness and swelling of mouth	Niacin, riboflavin, iron, and/or pyridoxine deficiency
Angular fissures, scars at corner of mouth	
Gums	
Spongy; swollen; bleed easily; redness	Vitamin C deficiency
Gingivitis	Vitamin A, niacin, riboflavin deficiency
Mouth	
Cheilosis, angular scars	Riboflavin, folic acid deficiency
Tongue	
Sores, swollen, scarlet, and raw	Folacin, niacin deficiency
Smooth with papillae (small projections)	Riboflavin, vitamin B_{12}, pyridoxine deficiency
Glossitis	Iron, zinc deficiency
Purplish color	Riboflavin deficiency
Taste	
Sense of taste diminished	Zinc deficiency
Teeth	
Gray-brown spots	Increased fluoride intake
Missing or erupting abnormally	Generally poor nutrition
Face	
Skin color loss, dark cheeks and eyes; enlarged parotid glands, scaling of skin around nostrils	Protein-energy deficiency; specifically niacin, riboflavin, and pyridoxine deficiencies
Pallor	Iron, folacin, vitamin B_{12} and vitamin C deficiencies
Hyperpigmentation	Niacin deficiency
Neck	
Thyroid enlargement	Iodine deficiency
Symptoms of hypothyroidism	
Nails	
Fragility, banding	Protein deficiency
Spoon-shaped	Iron deficiency

Table 7.5 (continued)

Physical Signs of Malnutrition

Signs	Possible causes
Skin	
Slow wound healing	Zinc deficiency
Psoriasis	Biotin deficiency
Scaliness	Biotin deficiency
Black and blue marks due to skin bleeding	Vitamin C and/or K deficiency
Dryness, mosaic, sandpaper feel, flakiness	Increased or decreased vitamin A
Swollen and dark	Niacin deficiency
Lack of fat under skin or bilateral edema	Protein-energy deficiency
Yellow colored	Carotene deficiency or excess
Cutaneous flushing	Niacin
Pallor	Iron, folic acid deficiencies
Gastrointestinal	
Anorexia, flatulence, diarrhea	Vitamin B_{12} deficiency
Muscular System	
Weakness	Phosphorus or potassium deficiency
Wasted appearance	Protein-energy deficiency
Calf tenderness; absent knee jerks	Thiamin deficiency
Peripheral neuropathy	Folacin, pyridoxine, pantothenic acid, phosphate, thiamin deficiencies
Muscle twitching	Magnesium or pyridoxine excess or deficiency
Muscle cramps	Chloride decreased, sodium deficiency
Muscle pain	Biotin deficiency
Skeletal System	
Demineralization of bone	Calcium, phosphorus, vitamin D deficiencies
Epiphyseal enlargement of leg and knee	Vitamin D deficiency
Bowed legs	Vitamin D deficiency
Nervous System	
Listlessness	Protein-energy deficiency
Loss of position and vibratory sense; decrease and loss of ankle and knee reflexes	Thiamin, vitamin B_{12} deficiencies
Seizures, memory impairment, and behavioral disturbances	Magnesium, zinc deficiencies
Peripheral neuropathy, dementia	Pyridoxine deficiency

Skin Integrity

The loss of skin elasticity and moisture and reduced feeling in susceptible areas place the elderly resident at risk for impaired skin integrity. Nutritional factors that contribute to skin breakdown include: protein deficiency, creating a negative nitrogen balance; anemia, inhibiting the formation of red blood cells; and dehydration, causing dry, fragile skin, which can result in an increase in the blood glucose level and slow the healing process. When conducting a nutrition audit, note the temperature and color of the skin. Hot skin may indicate increased blood flow due to inflammation or infection. Cool or cold skin with a white or pale color usually indicates decreased blood flow and impaired circulation. Wrinkled, withered, or dry skin is a sign of dehydration. Taut and shiny skin may indicate edema. When assessing a resident's skin, note that the presence of moisture contributes to the development of pressure ulcers. An incontinent resident is at risk due to the skin's increased exposure to bacteria and toxins in the urine and feces. Excessive perspiration also may render a resident at risk. Causes of excessive perspiration may be heavy clothing or bedding, or an elevated temperature. Breaks in the skin, as well as blemishes, rashes, lesions, and discolored areas, are warning signs of irritation or trauma and should also be noted. With advancing age comes decreased skin response to temperature, pain, and pressure. This affects the skin's elasticity and the healing process.[5]

Interview Summation

At the close of the interview, summarize the main points. Tell the resident how the information will be used, when to expect the next visit, and how to contact the dietary department. Tell the resident how often you will visit and the name of the dietetic technician or dietary manager, whom the resident or family can contact. Several visits and observations are needed to complete the MDS and the nutrition assessment. Family and staff members can provide information to help complete the assessment.

When the interview is completed, the registered dietitian reviews the medical record and completes the nutrition assessment. OBRA guidelines specify that care plans be developed in 21 days (7 days after the completion of the MDS). The following section presents standard protocols to help the registered dietitian complete the assessment.

Anthropometry

Anthropometry is the measurement of body size, weight, and proportions and is used to evaluate the nutritional status of residents. Low body weight, when associated with illness or injury, increases the risk of morbidity. Obesity is common among nonambulatory persons and residents whose caloric expenditure is low. The dietetic technician or dietary manager may collect preliminary information and begin the assessment, but the registered dietitian is responsible for the analysis and evaluation of the information to determine the nutritional status of each resident. The registered dietitian should ensure that the methods used to weigh and measure residents are reliable, since accurate height and weight data are imperative. Loss of height, for example, is an early indicator of osteoporosis. Measure and record height annually.

Standard Measures

STATURE

To obtain height on an ambulatory resident:

- Have person being measured wear minimum clothing so that posture can be clearly seen;
- Instruct person to stand tall, with bare heels as close together as possible, legs straight, arms at sides, shoulders relaxed, head erect, and eyes looking straight ahead;
- Have person take deep breath;
- Take measurement at point of person's maximum inspiration with your eyes at headboard level to avoid errors due to parallax;
- Record measurement to nearest 0.1 cm or 0.125 in; repeated measurements should agree within 1 cm or 0.5 in;
- Compare present measurement with previous stature measurement(s) and with reference tables or graphs to determine change and to aid with interpretation of measurements.[1]

HEIGHT

To estimate height of nonambulatory persons use one of the following methods:

1. The arm span measurement is roughly equal to the height of both men and women at maturity (within approximately 10%).[7] Span measurement is calculated as follows: with the upper extremities including the hands fully extended and parallel to the ground, measure the distance between the tip of one middle finger to the tip of the other middle finger. The span measurement remains constant in spite of decreasing height and is an acceptable alternate method for establishing the height.

2. Stature from knee height can be used to estimate the stature of an elderly person who is bedfast or chairbound or who has such spinal curvature that an accurate stature measurement cannot be obtained. Unlike stature, knee height changes little with increasing age. This estimated stature value can then be used in indexes when estimating basal energy expenditure with the Harris-Benedict equation. The computation of stature requires the person's knee height, age, and sex. One formula is used for men and another for women. The following formulas are used to compute stature:

$$\text{Men} = 64.19 - (0.04 \times \text{age}) + (2.02 \times \text{knee height})$$
$$\text{Women} = 84.88 - (0.24 \times \text{age}) + (1.83 \times \text{knee height})$$

In these equations, the knee height measurement is in centimeters (cm), and age is rounded to the nearest whole year. If knee height has been recorded in inches, multiply by 2.54 to convert it to centimeters. The estimated stature derived from the equation is in centimeters. If a stature estimate in inches is desired, the number derived from the equation is divided by 2.54.*

WEIGHT

The ambulatory resident can be weighed on an upright balance beam scale, but the spring-type bathroom scale should not be used because it is not accurate enough for clinical purposes. If the nonambulatory resident can sit, a movable wheelchair balance beam scale can be used. Bed scales are available for measuring the weight of the bedfast resident.

Standing measurement. To obtain an accurate standing weight:
■ Be familiar with use of instrument;
■ Calibrate scale to zero;
■ Weigh person at same time of day on the routine schedule and, if possible, by same staff person;
■ Weigh resident nude or in light underclothing, without shoes;
■ Position resident's feet over center of platform;
■ Adjust weights on balance beam, then read and accurately record measurement to nearest 0.25 lb or on a digital scale the reading should be to nearest 0.1 kg/lb;
■ Compare present measurement with previous weight measurement(s) and with reference tables or graphs to determine change and to aid with interpretation of measurements.

Seated or prone measurement. Suggestions for an accurate seated or prone measurement are:
■ For chair scale, position subject upright in center of chair, leaning on backrest.
■ Weigh resident and wheelchair, then weigh the wheelchair alone and subtract that weight.
■ For bed scale, position subject comfortably in center of sling.

A second measurement for either method must be taken to verify accuracy of weight.

Frequent checking and adjustment of the zero weight on the horizontal beam of the scale are necessary to ensure accuracy. The main and fractional sliding weights should be placed at their respective zero positions, and the zeroing weight should then be moved until the beam balances at zero. The accuracy of the scales should be checked with a set of standard weights or by a dealer of weights and measures at least two or three times a year.[1]

BODY FRAME SIZE

Following are two methods to estimate body frame size:
Wrist circumference size is determined by measuring the smallest part

---

* Adapted with permission of Ross Laboratories, Columbus, OH 43216, from *Nutritional Assessment of the Elderly Through Anthropometry,*[1] © 1984 Ross Laboratories.

of the wrist distal to the styloid process of the ulna and radius. Values are affected by variability of soft tissue. The r value is then determined by the following ratio and compared with the ranges in *Table 7.6*:

height (cm)/wrist circumference (cm)

Table 7.6

r Values for Frame Size

Men r value	Frame size	Women r value
≥10.4	Small	≥11.0
9.6 – 10.4	Medium	10.1 – 11.0
≤9.6	Large	≤10.1

Data from Grant J. *Handbook of Total Parenteral Nutrition*. Philadelphia, Pa: WB Saunders Co; 1980.

Elbow breadth is measured with the forearm upward at a 90-degree angle. The distance between the outer aspects of the two prominent bones on either side of the elbow is considered to be the elbow breadth. An elbow breadth less than the medium-frame values listed in *Table 7.7* indicates a small frame. An elbow breadth greater than those listed in Table 7.7 indicates a large frame.

Table 7.7

Elbow Breadth Measures for Medium-Size Frame

Women

Height in 1-in heels	Elbow breadth
4'10" – 4'11"	2-¼" – 2-½"
5'0" – 5'3"	2-¼" – 2-½"
5'4" – 5'7"	2-⅜" – 2-⅝"
5'8" – 5'11"	2-⅜" – 2-⅝"
6'0"	2-½" – 2-¾"

Men

Height in 1-in heels	Elbow breadth
5'2" – 5'3"	2-½" – 2-⅞"
5'4" – 5'7"	2-⅝" – 2-⅞"
5'8" – 5'11"	2-¾" – 3"
6'0" – 6'3"	2-¾" – 3-⅛"
6'4"	2-⅞" – 3-¼"

Adapted from Frisancho AR. *Am J Clin Nutr*. 1988; 37:311. Reprinted with permission.

MIDARM CIRCUMFERENCE AND TRICEPS SKINFOLD

Measurements of midarm circumference and triceps skinfold thickness can be used together to estimate body muscle mass by calculating the midarm muscle area.

The circumference of the upper arm is measured at its midpoint. To identify midpoint, the left arm is bent 90 degrees at the elbow, and the forearm is placed palm down across the middle of the body. The upper arm should be approximately parallel to the trunk. The midpoint is half the distance between the acromion and alecranor processes. Mark the skin at this point.

To obtain the midarm circumference, extend the left arm alongside the body with palm facing upward. Elevate the arm slightly at the elbow. Place the resident's hand through the insertion tape. Move the tape upward to the marked midpoint. The tape should be snug but not too tight. Repeat measurement. Successive measurements should agree with 0.5 cm. *Table 7.8* shows percentiles for midarm circumference.

Table 7.8

Percentiles for Midarm Circumference (in cm)

Age (y)	95%	50%	5%
Men			
65	37.8	31.9	26.7
70	37.2	31.3	26.0
75	36.6	30.7	25.4
80	36.0	30.1	24.8
85	35.3	29.4	24.2
90	34.7	28.8	23.5
Women			
65	37.0	30.5	25.3
70	36.6	30.2	24.9
75	36.3	29.8	24.6
80	35.9	29.5	24.2
85	35.6	29.1	23.9
90	35.2	28.9	23.5

Adapted with permission of Ross Laboratories, Columbus, OH 43216, from *Nutritional Assessment of the Elderly Through Anthropometry,* ©1984 Ross Laboratories.

To obtain the triceps skinfold measurement, have the resident lie on the right side with the right arm extended out from the body and the hand resting under the head. The trunk is in a straight line and the legs are slightly bent. The left arm rests along the trunk, palm down. The triceps skinfold thickness measurement is made on the back of the arm at the level of the marked midpoint. Grasp a double fold of skin and subcutaneous tissue between the thumb and index finger. Hold the skin while positioning the jaws of a skinfold caliper perpendicular to the fold. To read the caliper, bend down to avoid error due to parallax. Repeat measurements (successive measurements should agree within 3 mm) and compare with the values given in *Table 7.9* to obtain the resident's percentile.

Table 7.9

Percentiles for Triceps Skinfold Thickness (in mm)

Age (y)	95%	50%	5%
Men			
65	27.0	13.8	8.6
70	26.1	12.9	7.7
75	25.2	12.0	6.8
80	24.3	11.2	6.0
85	23.4	10.3	5.1
90	22.6	9.4	4.2
Women			
65	33.0	21.6	13.5
70	32.0	20.6	12.5
75	31.0	19.6	11.5
80	30.0	18.6	10.5
85	29.0	17.6	9.5
90	28.0	16.6	8.5

Adapted with permission of Ross Laboratories, Columbus, OH 43216, from *Nutritional Assessment of the Elderly Through Anthropometry*, ©1984 Ross Laboratories.

Table 7.10

Body Mass Index*†

Height inches	meters	45.3 (100)	49.90 (110)	54.43 (120)	58.97 (130)	63.50 (140)	68.04 (150)	72.57 (160)	77.11 (170)	81.65 (180)	86.18 (190)	90.72 (200)	95.25 (210)	99.79 (220)	104.33 (230)	108.86 (240)	113.40 (250)	117.93 (260)	122.47 (270)	127.01 (280)	131.54 (290)	136.08 (300)
															Weight kg (lb)							
55	1.397	23.24	25.56	27.89	30.21	32.54	34.86	37.19	39.51	41.84												
56	1.422	22.43	24.67	26.92	29.16	31.40	33.65	35.89	38.13	40.37	42.62											
57	1.448	21.64	23.80	25.96	28.13	30.29	32.46	34.62	36.79	38.95	41.12	43.28										
58	1.473	20.90	22.99	25.08	27.17	29.26	31.35	33.44	35.53	37.62	39.71	41.80	43.89									
59	1.498	20.20	22.22	24.24	26.26	28.28	30.29	32.32	34.33	36.35	38.37	40.39	42.41	44.43								
60	1.524	19.53	21.48	23.43	25.39	27.34	29.29	31.25	33.20	35.15	37.11	39.06	41.01	42.96	44.92	46.87	48.82	50.78	52.73	54.68	56.64	58.59
61	1.549	18.89	20.78	22.67	24.56	26.45	28.34	30.23	32.12	34.01	35.90	37.79	39.68	41.57	43.46	45.35	47.24	49.13	51.02	52.90	54.79	56.68
62	1.575	18.29	20.12	21.95	23.78	25.61	27.44	29.26	31.09	32.92	34.75	36.58	38.41	40.24	42.07	43.90	45.72	47.55	49.38	51.21	53.04	54.87
63	1.600	17.71	19.48	21.26	23.03	24.80	26.57	28.34	30.11	31.88	33.66	35.43	37.20	38.97	40.74	42.51	44.28	46.06	47.83	49.60	51.37	53.14
64	1.626	17.16	18.88	20.60	22.31	24.03	25.75	27.46	29.18	30.90	32.61	34.33	36.05	37.76	39.48	41.20	42.91	44.63	46.34	48.06	49.78	51.49
65	1.651	16.64	18.30	19.97	21.63	23.30	24.96	26.62	28.29	29.95	31.62	33.28	34.94	36.61	38.27	39.94	41.60	43.26	44.93	46.59	48.26	49.92
66	1.676	16.14	17.75	19.37	20.98	22.60	24.21	25.82	27.44	29.05	30.67	32.28	33.89	35.51	37.12	38.74	40.35	41.96	43.58	45.19	46.81	48.42
67	1.702	15.66	17.23	18.79	20.36	21.93	23.49	25.06	26.62	28.19	29.76	31.32	32.89	34.46	36.02	37.59	39.15	40.72	42.29	43.85	45.42	46.99
68	1.727	15.20	16.72	18.24	19.77	21.29	22.81	24.33	25.85	27.37	28.89	30.41	31.93	33.45	34.97	36.49	38.01	39.53	41.05	42.57	44.09	45.61
69	1.753	14.77	16.24	17.72	19.20	20.67	22.15	23.63	25.10	26.58	28.06	29.53	31.01	32.49	33.96	35.44	36.92	38.39	39.87	41.35	42.82	44.30
70	1.778	14.35	15.78	17.22	18.65	20.09	21.52	22.96	24.39	25.83	27.26	28.70	30.13	31.57	33.00	34.44	35.87	37.30	38.74	40.17	41.61	43.04
71	1.803		15.34	16.74	18.13	19.52	20.92	22.32	23.71	25.10	26.50	27.89	29.29	30.68	32.08	33.47	34.87	36.26	37.66	39.05	40.45	41.84
72	1.829		14.92	16.27	17.63	18.99	20.34	21.70	23.05	24.41	25.77	27.12	28.48	29.84	31.19	32.55	33.90	35.26	36.62	37.97	39.33	40.69
73	1.854		14.51	15.83	17.15	18.47	19.79	21.11	22.43	23.75	25.07	26.39	27.71	29.02	30.34	31.66	32.98	34.30	35.62	36.94	38.26	39.58
74	1.879		14.12	15.41	16.69	17.97	19.26	20.54	21.83	23.11	24.39	25.68	26.96	28.25	29.53	30.81	32.10	33.38	34.66	35.95	37.23	38.52
75	1.905			14.99	16.25	17.50	18.75	20.00	21.25	22.50	23.75	25.00	26.25	27.49	28.75	30.00	31.25	32.50	33.75	35.00	36.25	37.50
76	1.930			14.61	15.82	17.04	18.26	19.47	20.69	21.91	23.13	24.34	25.56	26.78	27.99	29.21	30.43	31.65	32.86	34.08	35.30	36.52

*From Bray GA, et al. Evaluation of the obese patient. I. An algorithm. JAMA. 1976; 235:1487. Copyright 1976, American Medical Association. Reprinted with permission.

†Expressed as weight (kg)/height (m)².

BODY MASS INDEX

Body mass index (BMI) is used as an indicator of body fatness and/ or ideal body weight. The BMI is a weight to height ratio composed of body weight (in kilograms) divided by the square of the height in meters, or weight/ height². Minimum survivable weight for humans is probably 50% to 55% of desirable body weight; the Committee on Diet and Health, 1989 states that a BMI of less than 24 is significant for people older than 65 years. The BMI is highly correlated with body fat, but increased lean body mass, or a large body frame, can also increase the BMI. It is generally agreed that a normally hydrated person with a BMI of 30 would be obese, and that a person with a BMI of more than 27 would be at major risk for obesity.[2]

The BMI table (*Table 7.10*) is not age-related because it does not consider the variable height loss with age. Thus, if your height decreases while your weight remains stable, your BMI increases, which may not be a true indication of nutritional status. It is recommended the midarm circumference be measured. This measure is highly correlated with the BMI (the Spearman rank correlation coefficient of midarm circumferences with BMI for the instutitionalized elderly is 0.69 for men and 0.89 for women). Low weight for height calculated as BMI, may indicate poor nutritional status.

AMPUTATION

For a resident who has suffered a loss of body parts, ideal or target weight must be adjusted. The following percentages can be used as a guide when calculating an adjusted weight (*Figure 7.1*). Entire arm, 6.5%; hand and forearm, 3.1%; hand, 0.8%; entire leg, 18.5%; above knee, 11.6%; below knee and foot, 7.1%; below knee, 5.3%; and foot, 1.8%.[8]

Figure 7.1

Percentage of Total Body Weight
Contributed by Individual Body Parts

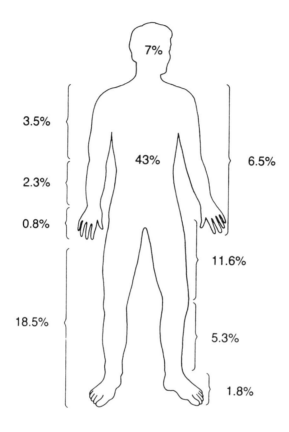

Adapted from Brunnstrom MA. *Clinical Kinesiology.* 3rd ed. Philadelphia, Pa: FA Davis; 1981. Reprinted with permission.

PARAPLEGICS AND QUADRIPLEGICS

To calculate the ideal body weight for residents who are paralyzed, first determine the ideal body weight and subtract these values from the original weight. The values depend on the degree of paralysis: for paraplegics, 5% to 10%; for quadriplegics, 10% to 15%.[6]

HEIGHT AND WEIGHT

Weight and body composition change with age. Weight tends to peak in the sixth decade, with a gradual decrease beyond the seventh decade. Shifts in body composition are noted and the proportion of body weight that is fat increases, averaging 30% of the total body weight in the elderly, as compared to 20% of the total body weight in younger people. *Table 7.11* presents the Metropolitan Life Insurance Company's height-weight tables,

Table 7.11

Establishing Ideal Weight Range: 1983 Height-Weight Charts*

Height	Small frame	Medium frame	Large frame
Men			
4′8″	116-122	119-129	127-137
4′9″	118-124	121-131	129-139
4′10″	120-126	123-133	130-141
4′11″	122-128	124-135	132-143
5′0″	124-130	127-137	134-145
5′1″	126-132	129-139	136-145
5′2″	128-134	131-141	138-150
5′3″	130-136	133-143	140-153
5′4″	132-138	135-145	142-156
5′5″	134-140	137-148	144-160
5′6″	136-142	139-151	146-164
5′7″	138-145	142-154	149-168
5′8″	140-148	145-157	152-172
5′9″	142-151	148-160	155-176
5′10″	144-154	151-163	158-180
5′11″	146-157	154-166	161-184
6′0″	149-160	157-170	164-188
6′1″	152-164	160-174	168-192
6′2″	155-168	164-178	172-197
6′3″	158-172	167-182	176-202
6′4″	162-176	171-187	181-207
Women			
4′5″	96-101	99-111	108-121
4′6″	94-103	101-113	110-123
4′7″	96-105	103-115	112-125
4′8″	98-107	105-117	114-127
4′9″	100-109	107-119	116-129
4′10″	102-111	109-121	118-131
4′11″	103-113	111-123	120-134
5′0″	104-115	113-126	122-137
5′1″	106-118	115-129	125-140
5′2″	108-121	118-132	128-143
5′3″	111-124	121-135	131-147
5′4″	114-127	124-138	134-151
5′5″	117-130	127-141	137-155
5′6″	120-133	130-144	140-159
5′7″	123-136	133-147	143-163
5′8″	126-139	136-150	146-167
5′9″	129-142	139-153	149-170
5′10″	132-145	142-156	152-173
5′11″	135-148	145-159	155-176
6′0″	138-151	148-162	158-179

*Weights at 25 to 59 based on lowest mortality. Weight in pounds according to frame (in indoor clothing weighing 3 lb, shoes with 1-in heels).

Courtesy of Metropolitan Life Insurance Company. Reprinted with permission.

Table 7.12

Average Weight of Americans Aged 65-94

Height (in)	Ages 65-69	Ages 70-74	Ages 75-79	Ages 80-84	Ages 85-89	Ages 90-94
Men						
61	128-156	125-153	123-151			
62	130-158	127-155	125-153	122-148		
63	131-161	129-157	127-155	122-150	120-146	
64	134-164	131-161	129-157	124-152	122-148	
65	136-166	134-164	130-160	127-155	125-153	117-143
66	139-169	137-167	133-163	130-158	128-156	120-146
67	140-172	140-170	136-166	132-162	130-160	122-150
68	143-175	142-174	139-169	135-165	133-163	126-154
69	147-179	146-178	142-174	139-169	137-167	130-158
70	150-184	148-182	146-178	143-175	140-172	134-164
71	155-189	152-186	149-183	148-180	144-176	139-169
72	159-195	156-190	154-188	153-187	148-182	
73	164-200	160-196	158-192			
Women						
58	120-146	112-138	111-135			
59	121-147	114-140	112-136	100-122	99-121	
60	122-148	116-142	113-139	106-130	102-124	
61	123-151	118-144	115-141	109-133	104-128	
62	125-153	121-147	118-144	112-136	108-132	107-131
63	127-155	123-151	121-147	115-141	112-136	107-131
64	130-158	126-154	123-151	119-145	115-141	108-132
65	132-162	130-158	126-154	122-150	120-146	112-136
66	136-166	132-162	128-157	126-154	124-152	116-142
67	140-170	136-166	131-161	130-158	128-156	
68	143-175	140-170				
69	148-180	144-176				

Adapted from Master AM, Laser RP, Beckman G. Tables of average weight and height of Americans aged 65 to 94 years. *JAMA.* 1960; 172:658. Copyright 1960, American Medical Association. Reprinted with permission.

and *Table 7.12* presents average weights and heights of white Americans aged 65 to 94. However, some elderly residents may have a target or usual weight that does not correlate with any table. An 85-year-old woman may never reach a weight of 100 lb, and an obese resident may never achieve an "ideal" weight. The important issue is achieving a stable weight over a period of 6 months or more that corresponds to an average daily intake of 75% or more of the individual resident's calorie requirement.

WEIGHT VARIANCES

When evaluating weight variances, it is important to determine if weight gain or loss was a result of recent surgery, or treatment initiated (eg, radiation). Weight variances can also occur when staff members fail to use correct procedures to weigh a resident or weigh at different times of the day. Significant weight loss should be reported to both the physician and the registered dietitian to ensure proper intervention. The important issue is the percentage of weight variance, rather than the amount in pounds. An obese woman who loses 3% per month is not at risk; however, an 80-lb woman who loses 3% is at risk. Significant weight loss that results in a condition change lasting 14 days or more triggers a new MDS.

EVALUATING THE SIGNIFICANCE OF WEIGHT LOSS

Determining the significance of weight loss as well as actual weight loss in pounds is specified in the OBRA requirements for participation in Medicare and Medicaid facilities, as shown in *Table 7.13*.

The formula to determine weight change is:

$$\text{Percentage weight change} = \frac{(\text{usual weight} - \text{actual weight})}{\text{usual weight}} \times 100$$

Table 7.13

Weight Loss

Time interval	Significant weight loss (%)	Severe weight loss (%)
1 wk	1.0 - 2.0	> 2.0
1 mo	5.0	> 5.0
3 mo	7.5	> 7.5
6 mo	10.0	>10.0

Calories and Fluid

The current Recommended Dietary Allowances (RDAs)[4] concluded that there are insufficient data to determine separate RDAs for people 70 years of age and older. While there is some evidence that the elderly have different requirements for some nutrients, for example, intestinal absorption, particularly of minerals, may actually be impaired. However, there is no evidence that an increased intake of nutrients above the RDAs is needed or that higher intakes will prevent the changes associated with aging.[4]

Caloric Requirements

A kilocaloric estimate should be completed for each resident. To estimate kilocalories, calculate the basal energy expenditure (BEE) as specified in *Tables 7.14* and *7.15* and multiply it by the activity factor and the injury factor (*Table 7.16*). The activity factor of a resident confined to bed is 1.2; it is 1.3 for a resident out of bed.

Table 7.14

Basal Energy Expenditure (BEE)*: Males

Weight

lb	kg	kcal	lb	kg	kcal
88.0	40	616	187.0	85	1235
90.2	41	630	189.2	86	1249
92.4	42	644	191.4	87	1263
94.6	43	658	193.6	88	1276
96.8	44	671	195.8	89	1290
99.0	45	685	198.0	90	1304
101.2	46	699	200.2	91	1318
103.4	47	713	202.4	92	1331
105.6	48	726	204.6	93	1345
107.8	49	740	206.8	94	1359
110.0	50	754	209.0	95	1373
112.2	51	768	211.2	96	1386
114.4	52	781	213.4	97	1400
116.6	53	795	215.6	98	1414
118.8	54	809	217.8	99	1428
121.0	55	823	220.0	100	1441
123.2	56	836	222.2	101	1455
125.4	57	850	224.4	102	1469
127.6	58	864	226.6	103	1483
129.8	59	878	228.8	104	1496
132.0	60	891	231.0	105	1510
134.2	61	905	233.2	106	1524
136.4	62	919	235.4	107	1538
138.6	63	933	237.6	108	1551
140.8	64	946	239.8	109	1565
143.0	65	960	242.0	110	1579
145.2	66	974	244.2	111	1593
147.4	67	988	246.4	112	1606
149.6	68	1001	248.6	113	1620
151.8	69	1015	250.8	114	1634
154.0	70	1029	253.0	115	1648
156.2	71	1043	255.2	116	1661
158.4	72	1056	257.4	117	1675
160.6	73	1070	259.6	118	1689
162.8	74	1084	261.8	119	1703
165.0	75	1098	264.0	120	1716
167.2	76	1111	266.2	121	1730
169.4	77	1125	268.4	122	1744
171.6	78	1139	270.6	123	1758
173.8	79	1153	272.8	124	1771
176.0	80	1166			
178.2	81	1180			
180.4	82	1194			
182.6	83	1208			
184.8	84	1221			

Height

ft in	in	cm	kcal
4' 7"	55	139.7	699
8	56	142.2	711
9	57	144.8	724
10	58	147.3	737
11	59	149.9	749
5' 0"	60	152.4	762
1	61	154.9	775
2	62	157.5	787
3	63	160.0	800
4	64	162.6	813
5' 5"	65	165.1	825
6	66	167.6	838
7	67	170.2	851
8	68	172.7	864
9	69	175.3	876
5' 10"	70	177.8	889
11	71	180.3	902
6' 0"	72	182.9	914
1	73	185.4	927
2	74	188.0	940
6' 3"	75	190.5	953
4	76	193.0	965
5	77	195.6	978
6	78	198.1	991
7	79	200.7	1003
6' 8"	80	203.2	1016
9	81	205.7	1029
10	82	208.3	1041
11	83	210.8	1054
7' 0"	84	213.4	1067

Age

yr	kcal	yr	kcal	yr	kcal
18	122	48	324	73	493
19	128	49	331	74	500
20	135	50	331	75	507
21	142	51	345	76	514
22	149	52	352	77	521
23	155	53	358	78	527
24	162	54	365	79	534
25	169	55	372	80	541
26	176	56	379	81	548
27	183	57	385	82	554
28	189	58	392	83	561
29	196	59	399	84	568
30	203	60	406	85	575
31	210	61	412	86	581
32	216	62	419	87	588
33	223	63	426	88	595
34	230	64	433	89	602
35	237	65	439	90	608
36	243	66	446	91	615
37	250	67	453	92	622
38	257	68	460	93	629
39	264	69	466	94	635
40	270	70	473	95	642
41	277	71	480	96	649
42	284	72	487	97	656
43	291				
44	297				
45	304				
46	311				
47	318				

How to use this table:

Step 1. Obtain weight, height, and age of male subject.

Step 2. BEE = weight kcal + height kcal − age kcal
Example: 70-kg, 178-cm, 45-year-old male
BEE = 1029 + 889 − 304
BEE = 1614

*Based on the Harris-Benedict equation: BEE = 66.47 + (13.75 × weight in kg) + (5.0 × height in cm) — (6.76 × age in y). Reference: Harris J, Benedict F. *A Biometric Study of Basal Metabolism in Man*. Washington, DC: Carnegie Institution; 1919: 40-44. Publication 279.

Adapted with permission from *Kansas Diet Manual*. ©1992 Kansas Dietetic Association.

Table 7.15

Basal Energy Expenditure (BEE)*: Females

Weight

lb	kg	kcal	lb	kg	kcal
77.0	35	990	176.0	80	1420
79.2	36	999	178.2	81	1429
81.4	37	1009	180.4	82	1439
83.6	38	1018	182.6	83	1449
85.8	39	1028	184.8	84	1458
88.0	40	1038	187.0	85	1468
90.2	41	1047	189.2	86	1477
92.4	42	1057	191.4	87	1487
94.6	43	1066	193.6	88	1496
96.8	44	1076	195.8	89	1506
99.0	45	1085	198.0	90	1516
101.2	46	1095	200.2	91	1525
103.4	47	1104	202.4	92	1535
105.6	48	1114	204.6	93	1544
107.8	49	1124	206.8	94	1554
110.0	50	1133	209.0	95	1563
112.2	51	1143	211.2	96	1573
114.4	52	1152	213.4	97	1582
116.6	53	1162	215.6	98	1592
118.8	54	1171	217.8	99	1602
121.0	55	1181	220.0	100	1611
123.2	56	1190	222.2	101	1621
125.4	57	1200	224.4	102	1630
127.6	58	1210	226.6	103	1640
129.8	59	1219	228.8	104	1649
132.0	60	1229	231.0	105	1659
134.2	61	1238	233.2	106	1668
136.4	62	1248	235.4	107	1678
138.6	63	1257	237.6	108	1688
140.8	64	1267	239.8	109	1697
143.0	65	1277	242.0	110	1707
145.2	66	1286	244.2	111	1716
147.4	67	1296	246.4	112	1726
149.6	68	1305	248.6	113	1735
151.8	69	1315	250.8	114	1745
154.0	70	1324	253.0	115	1755
156.2	71	1334	255.2	116	1764
158.4	72	1343	257.4	117	1774
160.6	73	1353	259.6	118	1783
162.8	74	1363	261.8	119	1793
165.0	75	1372			
167.2	76	1382			
169.4	77	1391			
171.6	78	1401			
173.8	79	1410			

Height

ft	in	in	cm	kcal
4'	0"	48	121.9	226
	1	49	124.5	230
	2	50	127.0	235
	3	51	129.5	240
	4	52	132.1	244
4'	5"	53	134.6	249
	6	54	137.2	254
	7	55	139.7	258
	8	56	142.2	263
	9	57	144.8	268
4'	10"	58	147.3	273
	11	59	149.9	277
5'	0"	60	152.4	282
	1	61	154.9	287
	2	62	157.5	291
5'	3"	63	160.0	296
	4	64	162.6	301
	5	65	165.1	305
	6	66	167.6	310
	7	67	170.2	315
5'	8"	68	172.7	320
	9	69	175.3	324
	10	70	177.8	329
	11	71	180.3	334
6	0	72	182.9	338

Age

yr	kcal	yr	kcal	yr	kcal
18	84	48	225	78	365
19	89	49	229	79	370
20	94	50	234	80	374
21	98	51	239	81	379
22	103	52	243	82	384
23	108	53	248	83	388
24	112	54	253	84	393
25	117	55	257	85	398
26	122	56	262	86	402
27	126	57	267	87	407
28	131	58	271	88	412
29	136	59	276	89	417
30	140	60	281	90	421
31	145	61	285	91	426
32	150	62	290	92	431
33	154	63	295	93	435
34	159	64	300	94	440
35	164	65	304	95	445
36	168	66	309	96	449
37	173	67	314	97	454
38	178	68	318	98	459
39	183	69	323	99	463
40	187	70	328	100	468
41	192	71	332	101	473
42	197	72	337	102	477
43	201	73	342		
44	206	74	346		
45	211	75	351		
46	215	76	356		
47	220	77	360		

How to use this table:

Step 1. Obtain weight, height, and age of female subject.

Step 2. BEE = weight kcal + height kcal – age kcal
Example: 55-kg, 163-cm, 45-year-old female
BEE = 1181 + 302 – 211
BEE = 1271

*Based on the Harris-Benedict equation: BEE = 655.10 + (9.56 × weight in kg) + (1.85 × height in cm) – (4.68 × age in y). Reference: Harris J, Benedict F. *A Biometric Study of Basal Metabolism in Man.* Washington, DC: Carnegie Institution; 1919: 40-44. Publication 279.

Table 7.16

Suggested Injury Factors

Surgery, minor	1.1	Pulmonary disease	1.3
Infection, mild*	1.2	PPN, TPN	1.23
Infection, moderate*	1.4	Liver disease	1.3
Infection, severe*	1.6	Traumas, skeletal	1.35
Cancer therapy	1.3	Head injury with steroids	1.6
AIDS	1.6	Blunt/bruise	1.3
Burns, 40%	1.5-1.8	Burns, 100%	1.8-2.0

*Use infection levels for pressure ulcers.

Chronic Respiratory Disease Requirements

Residents with chronic pulmonary disease present a different set of problems for the registered dietitian. Routine weights are not the only way to monitor nutritional status for the resident with chronic obstructive pulmonary disease (COPD), since weight loss may be masked with edema. Measurement of triceps skinfold and midarm circumference, and calculation of midarm muscle circumference to determine fat stores and muscle mass can be used along with biochemical indicators of nutritional status. To account for the goals of maintenance and restoration of lean body mass, the Harris-Benedict Equation is modified by specific numerical factors[1]:

Modified caloric requirement (men) =
$$(66.47 + 13.75W + 5.0H - 6.76A) \times F$$
Modified caloric requirement (women) =
$$(655.10 + 9.56W + 1.85H - 4.68A) \times F$$

Where W = weight (kg); H = height (cm); A = age (years); and F = factor for maintenance of lean body mass (1.0-1.2), for restoration of lean body mass, or for anabolism (1.4-1.6).[11]

Ventilator-Dependent Resident

Nutrient requirements for the stressed pulmonary resident[12]:
- For maintenance, 25 to 35 kcal/kg per day
- For anabolism, 45 kcal/kg per day
- For nitrogen, 0.2 g/kg per day (for amino acids, 1.5 g/kg per day)
- Lipid, 30% to 60% kcal

Protein Requirements

The protein content of the elderly body changes with age as muscle diminishes and body fat increases. Muscle protein turnover accounts for 30% of the turnover in young adults and only 20% of that in the elderly. Serum albumin levels also decrease in elderly people who consume diets with adequate protein.[10] Munro and Young recommend that 12% to 14% of the total calories consumed by the elderly be in the form of protein because decreased caloric intake may lead to decreased protein use. This necessitates increased protein intake.[10] Protein needs are based on the IBW (*Table 7.17*).

Table 7.17

Protein Needs

Condition	Albumin level	Protein requirement
Normal nutrition	3.5 g/dL	0.8 g/kg/d
Mild depletion	2.8–3.5 g/dL	1.0–1.2 g/kg/d
Moderate depletion	2.1–2.7 g/dL	1.2–1.5 g/kg/d
Severe depletion	2.1 g/dL	1.5–2.0 g/kg/d
COPD		100–125 g protein/d total

Fluid Requirements

Baseline fluid requirements are determined by multiplying the resident's body weight in kilograms by 30 mL (2.2 lb = 1 kg). These recommendations are not for residents with severe cardiac problems or with fluid restrictions.

In older adults, the water content of the body decreases from 60% of body weight and may fall to 45%. The elderly may have a blunted thirst sensation; even healthy elderly residents have reduced thirst after water deprivation. Meeting fluid needs is important since renal-concentrating capacity declines with age. When fluid intakes are limited, the risk of dehydration increases.

Constipation is common in the elderly and a decrease in fluid intake complicates this problem. Nursing facilities often increase the fiber content of the menus in an effort to reduce the constipation problems of the residents, but they often fail to promote adequate fluid consumption.

Reassessments

Nutrition assessments should be reviewed and updated quarterly or whenever the resident experiences a significant change in physical condition. Significant change means

- Deterioration in two or more ADLs or cognitive abilities appear permanent;

- Permanent loss of ability to ambulate freely or use the hands to grasp small objects;
- Deterioration in behavior, mood, or relationships that cannot improve unless staff intervenes;
- Deterioration in resident's health status;
- Marked or sudden improvement in resident's health status.

Under the OBRA guidelines, the health care team has a period of 14 days to evaluate and decide whether a condition change is "likely to be permanent."

An example of a significant change would be an unplanned or undesirable weight loss of 5% or greater in 1 month, 7.5% or greater in 3 months, and 10% or greater in 6 months. Pressure ulcers, fractures, surgery, or the initiation of chemotherapy or radiation are other examples. *Table 7.18* provides a basis for reviewing residents' current status related to their nutritional status. Adjustments in the care plan can be made based on the progress report.

Table 7.18

Nutrition Progress Report

Current diet: _____ **Fluid restriction** _____

Supplements: _____ Type _____ Frequency _____
        % Supplement accepted: _____

Food/fluid acceptance %:_____% Breakfast _____% Lunch _____% Dinner

Self-help device: Type _____ Syringe-fed _____ Spoon-fed _____

        ___ Difficulty chewing   ___ Difficulty swallowing

        Meal location: **Degree of assistance:**

        ___ Rehab dining room   ___ Partial assistance

        ___ Room   ___ Feeds self

        ___ Dining room   ___ Total assistance

IBW/acceptable: _____ lb   Current wt _____ lb   _____% gain   _____% loss

Fluid balance: _____ Normal   _____ Edema*   _____ Dehydrated   _____ Ascites

*Describe: _____

Skin condition: _____ Normal   _____ Red*   _____ Fragile*   _____ Pressure sore*   _____ stage

*Describe: _____

Bowel habits: _____ Normal   _____ Constipation   _____ Diarrhea, chronic

Pertinent clinical data:
Labs: Date _____   **New medication since last review:**
Hemoglobin _____   _____
Hematocrit _____   _____
BUN _____   _____
Albumin _____
Total protein _____   **Daily requirements:**
Fasting blood sugar _____   ___ Kilocalories
Potassium _____   ___ Protein
Other _____   ___ Fluid

Changes since last summary: _____
_____
_____

Progress toward goal: _____
_____
_____

_____ Quarterly   _____ Hospital return   _____ Condition change

Signature: _____ Date: _____

Resident: _____ Room no: _____
Adapted from MEP Healthcare Dietary Services Inc, Evansville, Ind. Reprinted with permission.

References

1. Chumlea WC, Roche A. *Nutritional Assessment of the Elderly Through Anthropometry.* Columbus, Ohio: Ross Laboratories; 1984.

2. Hiam RJ. *Indicators of Poor Nutritional Status in Older Persons.* Washington, DC: Nutrition Screening Initiative; 1991.

3. Grant A, deHoog S. *Nutritional Assessment and Support.* 4th ed. Seattle, Wash: Grant and deHoog; 1991.

4. National Research Council. *Recommended Dietary Allowances.* 10th ed. Washington, DC: National Academy Press; 1989.

5. Mead Johnson Enteral Nutritionals, Consultant Dietitians in Health Care Facilities Dietetic Practice Group. *Preventing Pressure Sores.* Evansville, Ind: Mead Johnson Enteral Nutritionals; 1989.

6. *Pocket Resource For Nutritional Assessment*; Chicago, Ill: Consultant Dietitians in Health Care Facilities Dietetic Practice Group; 1990.

7. Rossman I. *Clinical Geriatrics.* Philadelphia, Pa: JB Lippincott Co; 1979.

8. Wilkens K, ed. *Suggested Guidelines for Nutrition Care of Renal Patients.* Chicago, Ill: The American Dietetic Association; 1986.

9. Gersovitz M, Motil K, Munro HN, Scrimshaw NS, Young VR. Human protein requirements: assessment of the adequacy of the current recommended dietary allowance for dietary protein in elderly men and women. *Am J Clin Nutr.* 1982; 35:6–14.

10. Munro HN, Young VR. Metabolism and requirements. In: Caird FI, Exton-Smith AN, eds. *Metabolic and Nutritional Disorders in the Elderly.* Bristol, England: John Wright and Sons; 1980:13–25.

11. Askanazi J, Weissman C, Rosenbaum SH, et al. Nutrition and the respiratory system. *Crit Care Med.* 1982: 10:163–172.

12. Quality Assurance Committee, Dietitians in Critical Care Dietetic Practice Group. *Suggested Guidelines for Nutrition Management of the Critically Ill Patient. Process Criteria for Nutrition Assessment and Support of Selected Conditions.* Chicago, Ill: The American Dietetic Association; 1984.

8. WORKING WITH THE EATING-DISABLED OLDER ADULT

Quality of Life

Special Dimensions of Nursing Facilities

Autonomy

Eating Dependency

Positioning

Dining Room Atmosphere

Rehabilitation

8. WORKING WITH THE EATING-DISABLED OLDER ADULT

There is more to life than eating. But, considering the enjoyment received from dining with family and friends, it is difficult to find an activity in our lives that is equally important. Eating and mealtimes are essential elements of life; good food eaten in pleasant surroundings can enhance the quality of life.

The importance of food and mealtime does not change when a person is admitted to a nursing facility. This chapter reviews several aspects of mealtimes and assistance that have an impact on the eating-disabled older adult's quality of life.

Quality of Life

Mealtime is so much more than the simple intake of food. It is also time for pleasure. However, the many life-style changes that accompany the aging process can erode the older adult's dining pleasure as well as the ability to eat independently. As a person ages, physical changes may interfere with the ability to open packages or to use utensils. Biological changes, such as impaired hearing, impaired vision, and decreased sensory perception, also may interfere with consuming a well-balanced meal or participating in mealtime conversation. Chronic degenerative diseases often result in physical impairment. These physical impairments or disabilities result in loss of independent function—contributing to an individual's need for residential care and ultimately detracting from the quality of life.

Food and the atmosphere in which the food is served have an impact on quality of life for residents.[1-4] Dining atmosphere is one of the most crucial aspects of creating a pleasurable dining experience. A pleasant atmosphere consists of attractive physical surroundings, and more important, a climate of friendship and respect. Because of the social significance of mealtime, every effort should be taken to make each meal a positive experience. These concepts are so important that they were written into the Omnibus Budget Reconciliation Act (OBRA) regulations.[5] OBRA regulations emphasize enhancing quality of life for residents of nursing facilities.

Social considerations affect mealtime. People enjoy eating with family and friends. Seating arrangements should consider groupings that inspire social interaction. Caregivers should encourage interaction among diners and should themselves visit with residents during mealtimes. Residents will benefit from sharing mealtimes with like-minded persons of their own choosing. It is counterproductive to place confused, noisy, or behaviorally inappropriate residents with residents who are cognitively intact. Separate, equally furnished dining areas for disruptive residents and those engaged in restorative dining programs may be beneficial.

Special Dimensions of Nursing Facilities

The special dimensions and needs of nursing facility residents differentiate the approach to care in nursing facilities from those of other health care institutions, such as hospitals. Emotional and mental needs of residents often take precedence over their physical needs and significantly affect their quality of life.[6,7] For example, a resident placed on a strict diabetic diet may refuse to eat. However, the same resident may accept many of the diabetic restrictions when allowed to have some control over food choices, thus having an emotional and mental need met.

Autonomy

Overall health is influenced by one's sense of autonomy. Independence is developed over the years and becomes essential to mental health. The gradual deterioration in the body's physical condition that occurs with aging and chronic disease may limit this independence.[8] Even with physical changes, people are able to maintain personal autonomy if they perceive themselves as having some control over their lives. The example of the diabetic resident's acceptance of dietary restrictions when allowed to have some control over diet and food selection illustrates one aspect of personal autonomy.

Decisions often are made for residents because it is assumed that they are unable to make choices or express preferences. OBRA regulations empower residents with the right to make choices: expressing preferences regarding eating including the choice of mealtime, table companions, or food preferences. Having the opportunity to make choices and express preferences is one simple, yet important way to help maintain a high level of functional health.

Eating Dependency

Among adults older than 80 years of age, eating disabilities are common and increase with advancing age. Manual dexterity is a good predictor of independent eating skills. One study found loss of independent eating skills in 22% of people admitted to nursing facilities in 1988.[9] Another found that 40% of these residents required assistance or were fed enterally or parenterally.[10] Dependency status with respect to eating has been correlated with impaired mobility, impaired cognition, consumption of modified consistency diets, the presence of upper extremity dysfunction, absence of teeth or dentures, and behavioral indicators of abnormal oral motor status. Dependency in eating also was highly associated with mortality.[11]

In addition to the poor outcomes related to eating dependency, the costs of feeding assistance are considerable. The expenses of managing eating dependency have been estimated to represent a quarter of the cost of care for totally dependent individuals.[11]

Caregivers' attitudes toward residents directly affect mealtime performance. Staff members must be willing to lend assistance. The type and amount of assistance provided has a significant impact on a resident's ability to maintain independence. Residents who receive too much assistance may gradually lose the ability to eat independently. Therefore, it is important for the caregiver to be aware of residents' skill levels and to encourage them to be as independent as possible. Often new residents accept assistance more readily.

Residents benefit from an environment in which they are encouraged to function at their highest physical and mental levels. The importance of feeding oneself independently is vital for self-esteem. For residents who have temporarily lost the ability to eat independently, regaining independent eating skills enhances their sense of autonomy and self-esteem.

According to OBRA regulations, the residents have the right to expect that they should not physically deteriorate beyond what is normal for their diagnosed condition. The facility is required to maintain an environment to support independence in meal service.

Positioning

Positioning provides the key for maximizing eating independence. The ideal eating position begins with the use of a standard dining room chair with arm rests for support. The resident should sit in the chair with feet squarely on the floor, hips at a 90-degree angle at the back of the chair, head held upright and tilted slightly forward. The chair arm rests need to be positioned slightly under the table so that the resident's abdomen is close to the table. The distance from the plate to the mouth should be no more than 12 to 18 in. When additional support is needed to maintain this upright positioning, the resident can rest his or her elbows on the edge of the table.

For residents who are unable or refuse to transfer from a wheelchair to a standard dining room chair for meals, proper positioning in the wheelchair is of utmost importance. The table may need to be elevated to allow the wheelchair to slide under the edge. It is equally important for the resident in a wheelchair to be within 12 to 18 in of the plate. This requires the wheelchair to be locked into position with the resident's abdomen close to the table, and hips at a 90-degree angle. Solid support on the wheelchair seat and back in addition to foot support with foot rests or directly on the floor helps maintain the hips at the 90-degree angle.

The same positioning is beneficial for residents who must have meals while seated in a geri chair or in bed. Again, the hips are flexed at a 90-degree angle, and the head held upright with chin tilted slightly forward. Particularly beware not to allow the resident to tilt his or her head backward or too far forward, as either position can contribute to swallowing dysfunction or aspiration.

Dining Room Atmosphere

Dining atmosphere is one of the most crucial aspects of a pleasurable dining experience. The physical dining environment should be attractive and functional, and the room as homelike as possible. Tablecloths, napkins, flowers, and centerpieces go a long way toward setting the tone.

A simple dining room decor in light tones heightens vision, as does lighting that creates neither glare nor shadows. Using solid color, rather than patterns, in wall and floor treatments enhances visual perception and decreases the possibility of visual confusion.

Presentation of a few items on the table minimizes visual clutter and further enhances visual perception. Colorful dishes that contrast with the food enable the visually impaired to recognize items on the plate more easily. Tablecloths and placemats can provide additional contrast for the dishes and thereby help residents locate the dishes.

Distractions must be kept to a minimum. Television and radio should be off, although quiet background music may enhance the meal for those with unimpaired hearing. Traffic flow should be smooth to prevent distraction. A calm, relaxed mood with minimal noise is an ideal dining atmosphere.

Dressing for meals, combing one's hair, or fixing one's make-up all contribute to the anticipation of dining. For those who require them, dentures, glasses, or hearing aids are essential for mealtimes. At the table, the diner should be provided with a napkin that can be placed in the lap or tucked under the chin. To avoid the resident's looking infantile, a good napkin will replace the need for a bib.

Rehabilitation

Feeding oneself is basic to one's sense of autonomy. Therefore, it is important for the nursing facility staff to encourage and stimulate the residents' efforts toward independent eating. Encourage independence by offering appropriate levels of assistance, which is identified by careful assessment of each resident's eating ability. Once an independent eating level is identified, the resident should be allowed and encouraged to use existing skills.

Independent eating skills might include being able to hold a glass, direct the glass to the mouth, and drink. To maintain this skill, the resident always should be expected to drink independently. Direct care staff members may need to use verbal prompts to remind the resident to pick up the glass and drink, or may need to support the resident's hand to help hold the glass, as well as direct the glass to the mouth. This hand-over-hand assistance allows the resident to continue to go through the motions of picking up the glass and directing the glass to the mouth, permitting less chance of losing the ability.

Hand-over-hand assistance also can be used to help the resident eat with utensils. As the resident becomes stronger or more independent, the caregiver needs to withdraw assistance gradually. For instance, in lieu of hand-over-hand assistance, the resident might benefit from the assistance or support of the caregiver's hand under the forearm or at the elbow. Once the resident has food on the eating utensil, the caregiver can help direct the arm to the mouth by providing assistance at the resident's elbow. It is important not to provide more assistance than the resident needs. To increase independence, gradually reduce the amount of physical assistance while using only verbal prompts to provide the required direction.

Confused or forgetful residents who can move their hands to their mouths need to be involved in independent eating. These residents may need only verbal prompting, but they may need prompting at every step of the eating process. The prompts might follow this sequence: "[Resident's name], pick up your spoon. Scoop some potatoes with your spoon. Put the potatoes in your mouth. Swallow the potatoes." When verbal prompting is unsuccessful, the caregiver should try hand-over-hand assistance.

Repetition is an essential element of rehabilitation. The same is true for maintaining or regaining independent eating skills. Repetition and consistent approaches are necessary and may take several weeks to achieve progress. Encouraging the resident to use repetitive motions such as tooth brushing, face washing, hair combing, and shaving are helpful in the rehabilitation process.

Adaptive measures sometimes are necessary for the resident's comfort and independence. Adaptive equipment substitutes for motions lost because of disability. Before adaptive equipment and utensils are considered, the resident's posture and the way the resident is seated at the table must be addressed. Improved positioning at mealtime might eliminate the need for adaptive equipment.

A variety of adaptive equipment is available to facilitate independent eating. Large-handled flatware, nose cut-out glasses, inner lip plates, and large-handled travel mugs can be helpful. Consult an occupational therapist, if one is available, on the proper selection of adaptive equipment and utensils.

The entire health care team needs to be aware of residents' eating abilities as well as the impact of meal service on their quality of life.[12] A team approach is crucial in facilitating positive dining experiences. The physician, nurse, registered dietitian, speech language pathologist, occupational and physical therapists, social worker, dietary personnel, and the direct care staff, all play important roles. The care planning process using a team approach provides a means of communicating ways to promote, as well as maintain independent eating skills.

In summary this chapter points out the importance of each of the following elements concerning the eating-disabled older adult: quality of life, special dimensions of nursing facilities, autonomy, eating dependency, positioning, dining room atmosphere, and rehabilitation.

When you pay attention to all of these factors, you help the residents enjoy a positive dining experience, and as a result, maintain a higher quality of life.

References

1. Consultant Dietitians in Health Care Facilities Dietetic Practice Group. *Dining Skills: Practical Interventions for the Caregiver of the Eating-Disabled Older Adult.* Chicago, Ill: Consultant Dietitians in Health Care Facilities Dietetic Practice Group; 1992.

2. Deutschman M. Environmental setting and environmental competence.*Gerontol Geriatr Educ.* 1982; 2:237-242.

3. Langer EJ, Rodin J. The effects of choice and enhanced personal responsibility for the aged: a field experiment in an institutional setting. *J Personality Soc Psychol.* 1976;34:191-198.

4. Rozzini R, Beachetti A, Carabellese C, Inzoli M, Trabucchi M. Depression, life events and somatic symptoms. *Gerontologist.* 1988;28:229-232.

5. *Omnibus Budget Reconciliation Act of 1987. House of Representatives, 100th Congress Report.* Washington, DC: US Government Printing Office; 1987:100-391.

6. Jacobson HN. Nutrition and health related quality of life. In: *Food and Nutrition News.* Chicago, Ill.: National Livestock and Meat Board, Research and Nutrition Information Dept; 1989.

7. Speer M. Contributions of food service to quality of life in long term care facilities. *Top Clin Nutr.* 1989;4:19-26.

8. Davis BW, Mills EA, Mayewski P. Feeding with sensitivity: a workshop for nursing home staff. *J Nutr Educ.* 1989;21:82-84.

9. Applebaum RA, Wilson NL. Training needs for providing case management for the long term care client: lessons from the national channeling demonstration. *Gerontologist.* 1988;28:172-176.

10. Seibens H, Trupe E, Siebens A, et al. Correlates and consequences of eating dependency in institutional elderly. *J Am Geriatr Soc.* 1986;34:192-198.

11. Dwyer JT. *Screening Older Americans' Nutritional Health—Current Practices and Future Possibilities.* Washington, DC: Nutrition Screening Initiative; 1991.

12. Gilmore S, Russell CM. Factors affecting meal service in nursing facilities: employee's perceptions. *J Nutr Elderly.* 1992;11:1-3.

9. The Care Plan
A Team Approach

The Process

Developing a Resident Care Plan

Implementing the Plan

Monitoring and Evaluation

Documentation Guidelines

9. THE CARE PLAN: A TEAM APPROACH

The initial step in the care-planning process is the assessment, which identifies a resident's strengths, weaknesses, risk factors, and potential for improvement or anticipated decline. The assessment is used at the interdisciplinary team meeting to incorporate the problems into the plan of care.

Sections 1819 (b)(3), 1819 (e)(5), 1819 (f)(6)(B), 1919 (e)(5), and 1919 (f)(6)(B), of the Social Security Act, as amended by the Omnibus Budget Reconciliation Act of 1987 (OBRA), changed the total assessment process for all facilities certified to participate in the Medicare or Medicaid program.[1] This act states that facilities are "required to conduct a comprehensive, accurate, standardized, reproducible assessment" of each resident's ability to perform daily life functions. That excerpt from the Health Care Financing Administration's (HCFA's) *Resident Assessment Instrument (RAI) Training Manual and Resource Guide* perhaps best summarizes the requirements for resident assessment by nursing facilities, as specified in recent legislation.[2]

Extensive research and testing of the activities at various nursing facilities contributed to the development of the minimum data set (MDS) and the associated resident assessment protocols (RAPs). The MDS is considered to be the fundamental set of criteria needed to assess a person's functional status adequately. The total resident assessment instrument (RAI) consists of the MDS, triggers (RAP key, explained later), and the RAPs. The RAI provides information on the resident's condition, helps develop a plan of care, and is a means of tracking changes in the resident's status.

The Process

The flow of the resident assessment instrument–interdisciplinary care plan (RAI-ICP) information follows this sequence:
1. MDS
2. Worksheet/trigger legend
3. Problem/need list
4. Interdisciplinary care plan

MINIMUM DATA SET

This is used for the nursing facility resident assessment and care screening process. The registered dietitian must use several information sources to complete this section of the MDS, including:

- Observation of the resident
- Interview with the resident
- Interview with nurses and other nursing staff
- Discussion of resident's status with physician
- Discussion of resident's status with family member
- Discussion of resident's status with other facility staff
- Review of resident's records

The registered dietitian should examine the MDS thoroughly; there is much to be learned about the resident from this document. If the MDS is completed by a registered nurse (RN), the RN is responsible for signing the MDS. If the registered dietitian completes any section of the MDS, the registered dietitian is required to sign that section of the MDS. Although not required by HCFA, it is recommended that, when the MDS is completed by a person other than the registered dietitian, a progress note can indicate that the registered dietitian has reviewed it and either concurs with or questions what is documented in the MDS. If there are significant differences, a new MDS may be conducted. Areas of interest to review include: oral nutritional status, advanced directives (see last section of this chapter), changes in cognitive status, problems with communication or hearing, vision, changes in physical functioning, incontinence, failure to eat, wandering, lack of activity or exercise, diagnosis, health conditions, oral status, skin condition, medications, special treatments, and abnormal laboratory values. As a professional who is responsible for nutritional care, the registered dietitian has the responsibility to review the entire MDS and sign it with full name and date.

All completed MDS sheets are part of the resident's record. The first MDS always must remain with the chart. Others completed in the last 2 years must be easily retrievable on the active record. They are not necessarily in the resident's chart but are on the nursing unit or otherwise easily obtainable.

The MDS must be started within 4 days of admission and completed within 2 weeks of admission and at least annually thereafter. An MDS also must be completed promptly after significant physical or mental changes, and a review must be made no less than every 3 months. The interdisciplinary care plan meeting must be completed within 7 days following the signature on the MDS by the RN assessment coordinator. Significant changes can include:

- Deterioration in two or more activities of daily living (ADLs) or cognitive abilities that appear to be permanent (the health care team has 14 days to decide)
- Permanent loss of ability to ambulate freely or to use hands to grasp small objects

- Deterioration in behavior, mood, or relationships that cannot improve without staff intervention
- Deterioration in resident's health status (including weight loss)
- Marked or sudden improvement in resident's health status (eg, arm cast removal allows a resident to eat independently).

Upon readmission with a change in condition a full MDS is conducted. Upon readmission with no change in condition, a full MDS is not necessary.

RESIDENT ASSESSMENT PROTOCOL TRIGGER LEGEND

Once the MDS is completed, the trigger legend must be filled out to identify *automatic* or *potential* triggers. Automatic triggers direct the evaluator to go directly to the RAP instructions. Potential triggers direct the evaluator to go to the RAP instructions for more detailed trigger definitions.

RESIDENT ASSESSMENT PROTOCOL

This states the problem, describes it, and explains it if certain triggers are present. The RAP then lists guidelines for understanding the type of care that might be required. The RAP aids the interdisciplinary team in examining factors that may impede a resident's ability to achieve a certain goal or complicate treatment.

RESIDENT ASSESSMENT PROTOCOL SUMMARY

This form shows whether the interdisciplinary team is proceeding with a care plan intervention or has decided not to proceed. Documentation by discipline of problems, complications, and risk factors, or the need for referral to appropriate health professionals usually is found throughout the resident chart. The locations of this assessment information should be noted on the summary sheet so that others reviewing the data can readily find justification for the decision. Examples of instances when the team may not proceed to care planning from a triggered RAP:

- *Dehydration—resident does not consume all fluids provided.* The registered dietitian calculates fluid requirements and can justify that the resident does not need to consume all fluids provided: Resident calculated needs are 1200 mL or 30 mL/kg; resident receives 1800 mL daily. Resident shows no signs or symptoms of dehydration.
- *Nutrition—resident leaves more than 25% of foods uneaten.* The registered dietitian documents that this 100-lb, 90-year-old woman consumes only 50% of most meals. The registered dietitian calculates an average of 1800 to 2000 kcal in the regular diet. If the resident's basal energy expenditure (BEE) and total daily expenditure (TDE) have been calculated, the justification can note that this resident does not need the calories provided in the regular diet if no weight loss

is occurring. Small portions may be recommended. However, even if this is not addressed on the overall plan of care, it still must be addressed in the nutrition progress notes so that all members of the team are aware of the decreased overall intake.

- *Nutrition—mechanically altered diet.* The registered dietitian documents that a resident requires ground meat because he refuses to wear dentures after having them realigned and readjusted. The resident continues to request ground meat, consumes 75% of this food group, and shows no weight loss or signs of nutrition problems related to texture modification. Again, this would be covered in the progress notes, but progression to the care plan is not necessary.

During this phase of the process the team begins to develop the overall plan of care. Formal care plans must be developed within 21 days (7 days after completion of the MDS). The facility must develop a comprehensive care plan to address medical, nursing, and psychosocial needs identified in the assessment.

DISCHARGE PLANNING

This has not always been perceived as an important activity in the nursing facility; however, it is important for a number of reasons:

- When a resident is discharged to his or her home, written diet instructions are given for reference and reinforcement.
- Nutrition support programs may be contacted in advance and arrangements made for home-delivered meals.
- When a resident is discharged to a hospital or other nursing facility, the discharge summary can be a source of dietary information on nutrition status, explaining the degree of and the resident's response to nutrition intervention. This information can save the admitting facility time and prevent it from trying approaches that were previously unsuccessful. The nutrition discharge summary also can highlight a problem such as weight loss that might not be readily apparent to the admitting facility.
- Discharge planning can be an excellent opportunity to reinforce the principles of nutrition learned while the resident was in the facility. Residents returning to the home setting have a written reminder of the nutrition services offered by the facility.
- Discharge information may also facilitate the resident's adjustment to another environment. This should be a standard for providing health services.

A summary of the resident's nutritional status and problems while in one facility is valuable information for the facility that receives the resident and helps its dietitians develop an effective nutrition care plan much sooner than would be possible otherwise.[3] It also provides continuity of care and may, therefore, enhance the resident's quality of life.

Developing a Resident Care Plan

Resident care plans are implemented in nursing facilities to allow for an integrated approach involving not only the resident and facility staff, but also the resident's family or guardian and physician. The care plan for each resident includes an assessment of the resident's problems, documentation of measurable goals and approaches, and an evaluation of the outcome of the care provided. Every resident has strengths and weaknesses that must be considered. Goals of the care plan should be established with input from the resident when possible, recognizing the resident's priorities, rights, and needs.

The goal of resident care planning is to develop a course of action designed to maintain or return the resident to the best possible state of health. The dietitian develops the nutrition component using the interdisciplinary format in the facility.

In general, each resident's care plan should include:

- *Problems or needs* that must be addressed to attain and maintain the resident at the highest practicable physical, mental, and psychosocial well-being.
- *Realistic goals*, in terms of resident understanding, if possible. Goals must also be realistic and measurable, stated in terms of expected behaviors, changed as the resident's condition changes, have an anticipated date of completion or attainment, and designate responsibility.
- *Approaches* to solve problems and satisfy needs. The approaches must state what is to be done and by whom for each specified problem. In describing an approach, avoid words such as *encourage*, *understand*, or *reassure*. Instead use words that are specific and demonstrate action, such as "provide a cup with a large handle and teach resident how to use it to reach the goal of self-feeding and drinking."
- *An evaluation procedure*, because reviewing and reassessing the progress of the resident is an essential part of the care plan.
- *A discharge plan* developed in accordance with facility protocol.

The care plan is a part of each resident's medical record. It must be accessible to all who are involved in the care of the resident, the resident, and the resident's family or guardian. It is reviewed regularly to ensure that the approaches to improve or maintain the resident's state of health are effective.

Computer Programs

Because of the complexity of the resident assessment process, many nursing facilities computerize the MDS, RAPs, and other assessment data. Some software packages identify problems, produce prospective goals, and provide potential approaches once assessment data are entered. Computerization can assist in managing the process, but it cannot replace hands-on intervention by a concerned health care professional.

Desirable factors in a computerized program are:

- Changes in resident needs or conditions can be easily updated.
- Information in the database can be cross-referenced for interdisciplinary care planning.
- Predefined, standardized formats and care plan options can reduce lack of organization and save time.
- Manual updating or reproduction of the MDS/MDS+ form information is eliminated.
- All MDS forms are maintained in a history file and current MDS/MDS+ assessments are always on file.
- The care plan is quickly and easily produced using speed processing and the automatic incorporation of the RAPs and guidelines based on the resident's MDS assessment.
- Comparison reports are generated to ensure consistent and complete follow-up documentation.

Computers are a necessary adjunct to health care and can help health care professionals use their time effectively.

Implementing the Plan

One of the most effective methods for planning resident care is the interdisciplinary team conference. The interdisciplinary team conference offers an excellent opportunity for developing a coordinated plan for each resident. It allows each discipline to share its assessments and to gain greater understanding of the total needs of the resident. Much can be learned by carefully listening to and questioning other team members. Team cooperation is particularly important since implementing the goals often involves more than one discipline. For example, when one of the goals is weight reduction, the registered dietitian might develop a personalized diet plan and counsel the resident. The dietetic technician or dietary manager makes sure the food is served correctly and offers support to the resident. The activities director might devise activities to increase the resident's energy expenditure to include an exercise program commensurate with the resident's physical health, and the nursing staff provides support and ensures that extra food is not offered or brought in by visitors.

Nursing often is the appropriate discipline to chair the interdisciplinary team conference because of frequent contact with the other disciplines. It is desirable that all disciplines meet as a team at regularly scheduled intervals. The physician has ultimate responsibility for the health care of the resident by making the diagnoses and prescribing the medication, diet, and other treatments. He or she may be invited to the conference but generally is not asked to chair the team. The procedure followed by all disciplines should include:

- Collect data (information)
- Identify problems (needs)

■ Establish or review goals (objectives)
■ Determine plan (approaches)

Each discipline should come to the conference prepared to share its assessment data. Since the conference is usually prescheduled, the registered dietitian can prepare by collecting and updating the nutrition assessment data and developing tentative plans for dealing with the problem(s) identified.

The guidelines that follow are based on three major steps in care planning:

1. *Identify problems* through the use of a diet history, nutrition assessment, and the MDS. A problem is always a negative finding and should be stated behaviorally. The problem of the resident is a manifestation of or the result of a disease process or an injury. The problems are unique to the resident being reviewed.

2. *Establish resident-oriented goals* to resolve or control the problems identified. The goals for each discipline should be attainable within a reasonable time span. Goals should be realistic, resident-centered, and measurable. The goal belongs only to the resident and must not be a staff problem. The goal is usually a direct opposite of the problem.

3. *Develop specific approaches (plans)* to meet the goals. The approaches should be individualized, specific (eg, time span and responsible persons identified), practical, and understandable. Many goals established involve approaches (plans) from other disciplines to be attainable.[4]

Following the interdisciplinary team conference, the chair of the team follows up with written instructions. Many of these items will be suggestions and recommendations made by the disciplines, including the registered dietitian, at the conference. The dietary recommendations most often will be found in the progress summary of the assessment and will have been discussed during the team conference. The registered dietitian signs each care plan reviewed at the conference. If the registered dietitian is unable to attend the care conference, the recommendations should be disseminated at the interdisciplinary team conference by the dietetic designee, and the diet technician or dietetic supervisor signs the plan. The registered dietitian may review the plans later, initialing and dating the plans and progress notes.

The facility is ultimately responsible for the overall care of its residents including their nutrition care. The role of the registered dietitian is to identify problems and concerns. These procedures, therefore, ensure that recommendations made by the dietitian are included in the care plan if the registered dietitian cannot attend the conference.

Monitoring and Evaluation

The registered dietitian reviews the plans of care for residents at risk. Any problems with omission of nutritional goals or approaches to the care plan must be corrected immediately. Nutrition-related problems that might trigger such action include, but are not limited to, the following:

- Impaired skin integrity (making sure all areas with impairment are listed individually with the problem)
- Enteral or parenteral feeding regimens
- Unexplained weight changes (+/-)
- Renal dysfunction
- Unstable diabetes mellitus
- Increases in self-care deficits, especially quality of life issues such as rehabilitative feeding

Documentation and evaluation are integral parts of the process for the implementation of the goals and approaches established in the interdisciplinary team conference. Evaluating the care plan and determining whether goals have been met are both important. If the goals have not been accomplished, the following questions should be asked:

- Was this really a problem for the resident?
- Was the goal realistic?
- Was the goal stated in measurable terms?
- Did the approaches help the resident achieve the goals?
- Was the time frame realistic?
- Were the approaches realistic?
- Were the approaches carried out as listed?
- Was the appropriate discipline identified for each approach?

Answers to these questions should identify deficiencies in the plan and guide staff in correcting them. Remember to write care plans in the simplest terminology to ensure that all members of the team understand the plan. A written plan that is understood only by professionals is of limited value.[5]

The care plan is a permanent part of the legal medical record. Failure to identify and include a resident's nutrition needs in the care plan can be construed as professional neglect or lack of expertise on the part of the dietitian.

References

1. Department of Health and Human Services, Health Care Financing Administration. Section 4145, specifications of RAI for use in LTC facilities, appendix R. In: *State Operations Manual, Transmittal no. 241*. Baltimore, MD: Dept of Health and Human Services, Health Care Financing Administration; September 1990.
2. *Computerizing the Resident Assessment Instrument: A Special Report*. Washington, DC: American Health Care Association; September 1991.
3. Breeding C, Foster DM, Smith-Edge M. *The Consultant Dietitian: Developing Marketable Skills in Health Care*. New York, NY: Van Nostrand Reinhold; 1991.
4. Carson CH, Gerwick CL. *Guidelines for Nutrition Care*. Overland Park, Kan: Nutrition Education Center; 1988.
5. March C. *Care Plan Manual*. St Louis, Mo: Catholic Health Association of the United States; 1988.

Documentation Guidelines

Federal Interpretive Guideline 483.20(c) states that the accuracy of the assessment means the appropriate, qualified health professional correctly documents the resident's medical, functional, and psychosocial problems, and identifies the resident's strengths to maintain or improve medical status, functional abilities, and psychosocial status. The initial comprehensive assessment provides the baseline data for ongoing assessments of resident progress. The registered dietitian is the recognized professional for the nutrition care of the resident. Therefore, it is important that the registered dietitian who is employed on a part-time or consultant basis work closely with and train the dietetic technician or dietary manager to collect and record appropriate data for the completion of the resident comprehensive assessment, to prepare effective care plans, and to document any other pertinent resident information in the medical chart.

The assessment should paint a picture. Rather than "resident has dysphagia," it should explain that "resident has coughing, drooling, and pocketing." The assessment must be a comprehensive vehicle to track changes. It is the cornerstone for care planning. Following are guidelines for effective documentation:

- Use black ink as required on the MDS.
- Direct quotes from residents should be included and identified.
- State only facts; avoid phrases such as "appears to be" or "seems to be."
- When entering data on a form with blocks or spaces for specific data, complete all spaces. Draw a line through all unused blank spaces in a line.
- Use standard, legally valid abbreviations to save time (*Table 9.1*).
- Date all entries with month, day, year, and time.
- Sign all entries with full names and credentials.
- Do not obliterate anything on the record. If a mistake is made, line out the incorrect entry without rendering it illegible, sign and date the correction, then enter in the correct data. This is important because the medical record may be used as legal evidence.
- Document the indications for dietary interventions.
- When noting a referral of a return visit on a specific day, use the date, not the day of the week.
- Document all pertinent facts immediately.
- Do not back-date any medical record: it is illegal.
- Document teaching methods. Include what was taught, when the teaching occurred, what method was used, techniques used to ensure understanding of the material, and the resident's response.
- Document lack of resident compliance.
- Do not make uncomplimentary comments about the resident or a member of the resident's family in the medical record. Residents have access to charts.

Table 9.1

Commonly Used Medical Abbreviations

Abbreviation	Meaning	Abbreviation	Meaning
abd	abdomen	DVT	deep vein thrombosis
ac	before meals	Dx	diagnosis
ACVD	arteriosclerotic cardiovascular disease	ECG (EKG)	electrocardiogram
ad lib	as desired	ER	emergency room
ADD	attention deficit disorder	et	and
ADL	activities of daily living	ETOH	ethanol
adm	admitted or admission	Exam	examination
AKA	above knee amputation	eg	for example
ALb	albumin		
AM	morning	F	Fahrenheit
AMA	against medical advice	FBS	fasting blood sugar
amb	ambulatory	Fe	iron
amt	amount	ff	force fluids
APAP	acetaminophen	FH	family history
approx	approximately	fld	fluid
as tol	as tolerated	Fx	fracture
ASA	aspirin	F/C	Foley catheter
ASAP	as soon as possible		
ASBS	arteriosclerotic brain syndrome	GAS	generalized arteriosclerosis
		GB	gallbladder
ASHD	arteriosclerotic heart disease	GI	gastrointestinal
		glu	glucose
bid	twice daily	gm or g	gram
BKA	below knee amputation	GTT	glucose tolerance test
BM	bowel movement	gtt	drops
BP	blood pressure	g-tube	gastrostomy tube
BRP	bathroom privileges		
BUN	blood urea nitrogen	h or hr	hour(s)
		H₂O	water
c̄	with	Hct	hematocrit
C	centigrade, Celsius	HCTZ	hydrochlorothiazide
CA	cancer	HCVD	hypertensive cardiovascular disease
Ca	calcium		
CAD	coronary artery disease	Hgb	hemoglobin
cal	calorie	hs or HS	hour of sleep
cap	capsule	HTN	hypertension
CBC	complete blood count	Hx	history
CBR	complete bed rest	hyper-	above, excessive
CC	chief complaint	hypo-	less than, below
cc	cubic centimeter		
CCU	cardiac care unit	I & O	intake and output
CHF	congestive heart failure	IDDM	insulin dependent diabetes mellitus
CHO	carbohydrate		
Chol	cholesterol	IM	intramuscular
CNS	central nervous system	-itis	inflammation of
COPD	chronic obstructive pulmonary disease	IV	intravenous
CP	cerebral palsy	j tube	jejostomy tube
CVA	cerebrovascular accident (stroke)	K	potassium
CVD	cardiovascular disease		
CVI	cerebrovascular insufficiency	kg	kilogram
C/O	complains of		
		L	liter
DAT	diet as tolerated	lab	laboratory
DC	discontinue	lb	pound
DJD	degenerative joint disease	liq	liquid
DM	diabetes mellitus	lt or L	left
DON	director of nursing		

TABLE 9.1 (continued)

Commonly Used Medical Abbreviations

Abbreviation	Meaning	Abbreviation	Meaning
MAOI	monoamine oxidase inhibitor	q	every
MCT	medium-chain triglyceride	q4h	every 4 hours
meds	medication	qd	every day
meq or mEq	milliequivalent (23 mg Na = 1 mEq)	qh	every hour
		qhs	every night at bed
mg	milligram	qid	4 times daily
MI	myocardial infarction (heart attack)	qld	every other day
		qt	quarts
min	minute(s)		
mL	milliliter	RBC	red blood cell
mod	moderate	re	regarding
MOM	milk of magnesia		
		s̄	without
mOsm	milliosmole	SOB	shortness of breath
MS	multiple sclerosis	soln	solution
		SOS	if necessary
N & V	nausea and vomiting	spec	specimen
Na	sodium	SS	soap suds
neg	negative	stat	immediately or at once
NG tube	nasogastric tube	S/P	status post
NIDDM	non-insulin-dependent diabetes mellitus	T	tablespoon
NKA	no known allergies	tab	tablet
NKFA	no known food allergies	temp	temperature
nl	normal	TG	triglycerides
noc	night	TIA	transcient ischemic attacks (small strokes)
NPO	nothing by mouth		
NSAI	nonsteroidal anti-inflammatory	tid	three times daily
		TLC	total lymphocyte count
n/c	no complaint	TPR	temperature, pulse, respiration
N/V	nausea/vomiting	T Pro	total protein
		tsp	teaspoon
O₂	oxygen		
OBS	organic brain syndrome	URI	upper respiratory infection
od	once a day	UTI	urinary tract infection
OD	overdose		
OD	right eye	via	by way of
OOB	out of bed	VO	verbal order
OS	left eye	VS	vital signs
OU	both eyes		
oz	ounce	WBC	white blood count
		wk	week
pc	after meals	WNL	within normal limits
PEM	protein-energy malnutrition	wt	weight
PM	afternoon	w/c	wheelchair
po	by mouth (per os)		
postop	postoperative, meaning after surgery	x	times
preop	preoperative, meaning before surgery	yr or y	year
prep	preparation	Zn	zinc
prn	as necessary		
pt	pint	–	negative
Pt	patient	+	positive
PUD	peptic ulcer disease	>	greater than
PVI, PVD	peripheral vascular insufficiency or disease	<	less than
		↓	low, decreased
pwd	powder	↑	high, elevated
PT	physical therapy	°	degree

- Any discussions of problems, concerns, and so forth with the resident, the resident's family, or another member of the health care team should be recorded.
- Do not criticize prior care or the incompleteness of the record keeping of other health care professionals in the medical record.
- Be complete, accurate, legible, informative, and timely.

Finally, keep in mind that "If it's not recorded, it's not done or it didn't happen."

Advance Directives

An adult resident of a nursing facility who has the capacity to make personal decisions has the right to participate in decisions concerning his or her health care and medical treatment. An advance directive is a written instrument, such as a living will or life-prolonging procedure declaration, and an appointment of a health care representative and a power of attorney for health care purposes. These advance directives are established under state law and relate to the provision of medical care when a resident is incapacitated.

When a person is admitted to a nursing facility, the facility must provide the resident with information concerning advance directives to make sure that the resident understands his or her rights by law to make decisions concerning medical care. These rights may include the right to accept or refuse medical or surgical treatment and the right to formulate advance directives. The information should include a statement advising the resident of the facility's policy of respecting and honoring resident rights.

Signed copies of advance directives should be kept in the chart and on file. The attending physician should be apprised of the signed documents. A resident may revoke any advance directive at any time, without regard to mental or physical condition. A revocation is effective upon its communication to the attending physician or to any other health care provider by the declarant or by a witness to the revocation. A revocation of an advance directive is placed with the facility's original document.

The registered dietitian should be aware of the resident's advance directive procedures. These documents guide the registered dietitian in making recommendations for supportive care such as enteral or parenteral nutrition.

INDEX

213